1,000,000 Books

are available to read at

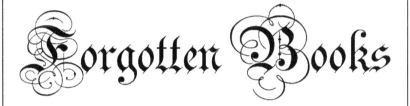

www.ForgottenBooks.com

Read online
Download PDF
Purchase in print

ISBN 978-1-332-86314-3
PIBN 10266458

This book is a reproduction of an important historical work. Forgotten Books uses
state-of-the-art technology to digitally reconstruct the work, preserving the original format
whilst repairing imperfections present in the aged copy. In rare cases, an imperfection in
the original, such as a blemish or missing page, may be replicated in our edition. We do,
however, repair the vast majority of imperfections successfully; any imperfections that
remain are intentionally left to preserve the state of such historical works.

Forgotten Books is a registered trademark of FB &c Ltd.
Copyright © 2018 FB &c Ltd.
FB &c Ltd, Dalton House, 60 Windsor Avenue, London, SW19 2RR.
Company number 08720141. Registered in England and Wales.

For support please visit www.forgottenbooks.com

1 MONTH OF
FREE
READING

at

www.ForgottenBooks.com

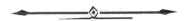

By purchasing this book you are eligible for one month membership to ForgottenBooks.com, giving you unlimited access to our entire collection of over 1,000,000 titles via our web site and mobile apps.

To claim your free month visit:

www.forgottenbooks.com/free266458

* Offer is valid for 45 days from date of purchase. Terms and conditions apply.

English
Français
Deutsche
Italiano
Español
Português

www.forgottenbooks.com

Mythology Photography **Fiction**
Fishing Christianity **Art** Cooking
Essays Buddhism Freemasonry
Medicine **Biology** Music **Ancient**
Egypt Evolution Carpentry Physics
Dance Geology **Mathematics** Fitness
Shakespeare **Folklore** Yoga Marketing
Confidence Immortality Biographies
Poetry **Psychology** Witchcraft
Electronics Chemistry History **Law**
Accounting **Philosophy** Anthropology
Alchemy Drama Quantum Mechanics
Atheism Sexual Health **Ancient History**
Entrepreneurship Languages Sport
Paleontology Needlework Islam
Metaphysics Investment Archaeology
Parenting Statistics Criminology
Motivational

Historic, archived document

Do not assume content reflects current
scientific knowledge, policies, or practice

U. S. DEPARTMENT OF AGRICULTURE.

BUREAU OF PLANT INDUSTRY—BULLETIN NO. 129.

B. T. GALLOWAY, *Chief of Bureau.*

BARIUM, A CAUSE OF THE LOCO-WEED DISEASE.

BY

ALBERT C. CRAWFORD,

PHARMACOLOGIST, POISONOUS-PLANT INVESTIGATIONS.

ISSUED AUGUST 22, 1908.

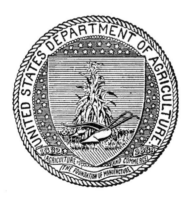

WASHINGTON:

GOVERNMENT PRINTING OFFICE.

1908.

BUREAU OF PLANT INDUSTRY.

Physiologist and Pathologist, and Chief of Bureau, Beverly T. Galloway.
Physiologist and Pathologist, and Assistant Chief of Bureau, Albert F. Woods.
Laboratory of Plant Pathology, Erwin F. Smith, Pathologist in Charge.
Investigations of Diseases of Fruits, Merton B. Waite, Pathologist in Charge.
Laboratory of Forest Pathology, Haven Metcalf, Pathologist in Charge.
Cotton and Truck Diseases and Plant Disease Survey, William A. Orton, Pathologist in Charge.
Plant Life History Investigations, Walter T. Swingle, Physiologist in Charge.
Cotton Breeding Investigations, Archibald D. Shamel and Daniel N. Shoemaker, Physiologists in Charge.
Tobacco Investigations, Archibald D. Shamel, Wightman W. Garner, and Ernest H. Mathewson, in Charge.
Corn Investigations, Charles P. Hartley, Physiologist in Charge.
Alkali and Drought Resistant Plant Breeding Investigations, Thomas H. Kearney, Physiologist in Charge.
Soil Bacteriology and Water Purification Investigations, Karl F. Kellerman, Physiologist in Charge.
Bionomic Investigations of Tropical and Subtropical Plants, Orator F. Cook, Bionomist in Charge.
Drug and Poisonous Plant Investigations and Tea Culture Investigations, Rodney H. True, Physiologist in Charge.
Physical Laboratory, Lyman J. Briggs, Physicist in Charge.
Crop Technology and Fiber Plant Investigations, Nathan A. Cobb, Crop Technologist in Charge.
Taxonomic and Range Investigations, Frederick V. Coville, Botanist in Charge.
Farm Management Investigations, William J. Spillman, Agriculturist in Charge.
Grain Investigations, Mark Alfred Carleton, Cerealist in Charge.
Arlington Experimental Farm, Lee C. Corbett, Horticulturist in Charge.
Vegetable Testing Gardens, William W. Tracy, sr., Superintendent.
Sugar-Beet Investigations, Charles O. Townsend, Physiologist in Charge.
Western Agricultural Extension Investigations, Carl S. Scofield, Agriculturist in Charge.
Dry-Land Agriculture Investigations, E. Channing Chilcott, Agriculturist in Charge.
Pomological Collections, Gustavus B. Brackett, Pomologist in Charge.
Field Investigations in Pomology, William A. Taylor and G. Harold Powell, Pomologists in Charge.
Experimental Gardens and Grounds, Edward M. Byrnes, Superintendent.
Foreign Seed and Plant Introduction, David Fairchild, Agricultural Explorer in Charge.
Forage Crop Investigations, Charles V. Piper, Agrostologist in Charge.
Seed Laboratory, Edgar Brown, Botanist in Charge.
Grain Standardization, John D. Shanahan, Crop Technologist in Charge.
Subtropical Laboratory and Garden, Miami, Fla., Ernst A. Bessey, Pathologist in Charge.
Plant Introduction Garden, Chico, Cal., W. W. Tracy, jr., Assistant Botanist in Charge.
South Texas Garden, Brownsville, Tex., Edward C. Green, Pomologist in Charge.
Farmers' Cooperative Demonstration Work, Seaman A. Knapp, Special Agent in Charge.
Seed Distribution (Directed by Chief of Bureau), Lisle Morrison, Assistant in General Charge.

Editor, J. E. Rockwell.
Chief Clerk, James E. Jones.

POISONOUS-PLANT INVESTIGATIONS.

SCIENTIFIC STAFF.

Rodney H. True, *Physiologist in Charge.*

C. Dwight Marsh, *Expert in Charge of Field Investigations.*
Albert C. Crawford, *Pharmacologist.*
Arthur B. Clawson, *Expert in Field Investigations.*
Ivar Tidestrom, *Assistant Botanist, in Cooperation with Forest Service.*

129
2

LETTER OF TRANSMITTAL.

U. S. Department of Agriculture,
Bureau of Plant Industry,
Office of the Chief,
Washington, D. C., April 10, 1908.

Sir: I have the honor to transmit herewith the manuscript of a technical bulletin entitled " Barium, a Cause of the Loco-Weed Disease," prepared by Dr. A. C. Crawford, Pharmacologist, under the direction of Dr. Rodney H. True, Physiologist in Charge of Poisonous-Plant Investigations, and to recommend that it be published as Bulletin No. 129 of the series of this Bureau.

For many years the stockmen in many parts of the West have reported disastrous consequences following the eating of so-called loco weeds characteristic of the regions involved. While many have doubted any causal relation between the plants in question and the stock losses, the reality of the damage has remained and has seemed to require a thoroughgoing sifting of the evidence concerning the part played by the plants. Accordingly, in the spring of 1905 a station for the experimental study of the problem was established at Hugo, Colo., in charge of Dr. C. Dwight Marsh, Expert, in cooperation with the Colorado Agricultural Experiment Station. Later a further feeding experiment was undertaken at Imperial, Nebr., in cooperation with the Nebraska Agricultural Experiment Station. Parallel with the feeding work in the field, laboratory work, designed to test under laboratory conditions the poisonous action of the plants from given areas, was undertaken at Washington by Dr. A. C. Crawford, Pharmacologist. A further phase of his part of the work was an attempt to ascertain the nature of such poisonous substance or substances as might occur in the loco plants.

In both of these lines of work Doctor Crawford has been successful, and the technical results of his work are here collected.

Respectfully,

B. T. Galloway,
Chief of Bureau.

Hon. James Wilson,
Secretary of Agriculture.

A scientific understanding of the so-called loco-weed disease has been demanded and sought after for several decades for most practical purposes, but, in spite of the great amount of attention which this problem has received, no general agreement has been found among the results obtained. The field investigations have given such contradictory evidence that until the Bureau of Plant Industry of the Department of Agriculture turned its attention to the matter the whole subject of the loco disease was regarded by many as a kind of delusion and the existence of a distinct entity was freely doubted. Not only did this confusion characterize the field aspect of the matter, but the situation viewed from the standpoint of laboratory study was also much obscured. Some investigators claimed to have separated poisonous substances of various sorts from the loco weeds, while others of equal scientific standing denied the presence of any poisonous substance in the plants under general suspicion—the so-called loco weeds.

In view of the great seriousness of the loco situation from the standpoint of the stock interests, an active campaign both in the line of feeding experiments in the field and laboratory study at Washington was undertaken by the Office of Poisonous-Plant Investigations of the Bureau of Plant Industry.

The feeding experiments carried out at Hugo, Colo., in cooperation with the Colorado Agricultural Experiment Station, before the close of the first season developed evidence that there was in reality such a thing as a loco disease. The investigator in charge was enabled to describe the disease in its most important manifestations and made it possible to sift the facts from the large number of contradictory statements in the literature.

The laboratory work, undertaken and carried on simultaneously, consisted of a pharmacological study, under laboratory conditions and with the usual laboratory subjects, of the action of plant material sent in from the field. The acute phase of loco-weed poisoning, as well as a more prolonged type of the disease, was studied. In plants found in this preliminary feeding to be harmful, the poisonous principle was sought, with the very striking results fully described in this paper. The demonstration of the presence of barium in the plants was followed by barium feeding, with the production of symptoms which agreed with those produced in the laboratory with loco extracts and in the field experiments with the loco plants as seen growing on the range. By comparing these laboratory results with those produced in connection with the field work, it became possible to sift the wheat from the chaff in the mass of contradictory evidence detailed in the literature of this subject.

The practical importance of the discovery of the true nature of the active poisonous principle of the loco weeds is very great. It not only sheds light on the loco situation and enables one to explain many hitherto inexplicable things, but it also adds much to our knowledge of barium in its medical bearings. It opens up most important problems concerning the soils and the relation of the flora to them. It should be borne in mind that although barium is shown to be chiefly responsible for the poisonous properties of loco weeds in eastern Colorado, it is entirely possible that in other regions other substances may be equally or even more significant. This discovery also seems likely to provide a basis for a rational treatment of locoed stock. Unfortunately, the discovery of the fact that barium is the poisonous constituent of loco weeds came too late to aid in the search for remedial measures on the range during the period covered by this report, but those empirically arrived at have received additional support from these laboratory results.

Thus the work in field and laboratory, undertaken after repeated attempts and discouraging failures by others, has yielded results to persistent scientific research and promises practical aid to the now suffering live-stock interests. The results of the laboratory work are presented in this bulletin.

RODNEY H. TRUE,
Physiologist in Charge.

CONTENTS.

BARIUM, A CAUSE OF THE LOCO-WEED DISEASE.

GEOGRAPHICAL DISTRIBUTION OF THE LOCO-WEED DISEASE AND ALLIED CONDITIONS.

In our Western States there is a marked annual loss of stock due to various causes. Some of these animals die in a condition known as " locoed," a term derived from the Spanish word " loco," meaning foolish or crazy.

This disorder extends from Montana to Texas and Mexico, and from Kansas and Nebraska to California.[a]

In 1898 the United States Department of Agriculture sent out, under the immediate direction of Mr. V. K. Chesnut, a request for information concerning the ravages of the loco disease. It was found that in the ten States of California, Colorado, Kansas, Montana, Nebraska, New Mexico, North Dakota, Oklahoma, Texas, and Wyoming the loss in 1898 was $144,850. Of this amount, $117,300 was attributed to Colorado alone; in fact, the disorder spread so that this State expended more than $200,000 in two years and over $425,000 in a period of nine years in attempts to eradicate the loco plants, the supposed cause of the trouble.[b]

The loss in one area of 35 by 120 miles in southwestern Kansas amounted to 25,000 cattle in 1883.[c] This loss in stock has been so great that the raising of horses has of necessity been abandoned in certain areas on account of the prevalence of these loco weeds.

It is difficult to obtain accurate data, as the ranchmen believe that any information as to the prevalence of the disorder would interfere with the value of their stock.[d]

Dr. James Fletcher, of the Central Experimental Farm, Ottawa, Canada, testified before the Select Standing Committee on Agri-

---

[a] Stalker, M. The "Loco" Plant and Its Effect on Animals. Bur. Animal Industry, 3d Ann. Rept. (1886), p. 271. 1887.

[b] Bur. Animal Industry, 6th and 7th Ann. Repts. (1889 and 1890). p. 272. 1891.

[c] Day, M. G. Loco-Weed. In F. P. Foster's Reference-Book of Practical Therapeutics, vol. 1, p. 587. 1896.

[d] O'Brine, D. Progress Bulletin on the Loco and Larkspur. Colo. State Agric. Coll. Bul. 25, p. 18. 1893.

9

culture and Colonization that he had never seen a case in the North-west of a Canadian bred animal being locoed, although the loco plants were prevalent. He explained this absence of loco disease by the abundance of grass on the range, because of which the animals do not acquire the habit of eating loco plants.[a] Cases have been reported, however, in Manitoba.[b]

PLANTS ASSOCIATED WITH THE LOCOED CONDITION.

The condition known as " locoed " is popularly believed to be due to eating various plants, especially the members of the Astragalus and Aragallus genera of the Leguminosæ, or pea family, but particularly to *Astragalus mollissimus* and *Aragallus lamberti.* These plants have therefore received the name " loco plants," [c] or crazy weed. But others, as *Astragalus mortoni,*[d] *A. hornii, A. lentiginosus, A. pattersoni,*[e] *A. nuttallianus, A. missouriensis, A. lotiflorus, A. bisulcatus, A. haydenianus,*[f] *A. tridactylicus,*[g] *Crotalaria sagittalis, Lotus americanus,*[h] *Sophora sericea, Caprioides aureum, Aragallus deflexa,*[i] *A. campestris,*[j] *A. lagopus,*[k] *Malvastrum coccineum, Amaranthus graecizans,* and *Rhamnus lanceolata,* are considered by some as loco plants.[l] In other places *Stipa vaseyi, Leucocrinum montanum, Fritillaria pudica, Zygadenus elegans,*[m] and even species of Delphinium are considered loco plants, so widely has this name been used.

In Mexico the term " locoed " embraces a condition due to the action of *Cannabis sativa* and various members of the nightshade family. This term has been much abused and has been made to embrace many groups of symptoms. In fact, if an animal dies while

---

[a] Fletcher, J. Evidence Before the Select Standing Committee on Agriculture and Colonization. Ottawa, 1905, p. 53.

[b] Fletcher, J. Experimental Farms Reports for 1892, p. 148. 1893.

[c] Sayre, L. E. Loco Weed. Amer. Vet. Rev., vol. 11, p. 555. 1887.—Stalker, M. The "Loco" Plant and Its Effect on Animals. Bur. Animal Industry, 3d Ann. Report. (1886), p. 271. 1887.

[d] Eastwood, A. The Loco Weeds. Zoe, vol. 3, p. 53. 1892.

[e] Chesnut, V. K. Preliminary Catalogue of Plants Poisonous to Stock. Bur. Animal Industry, 15th Ann. Rept. (1898), p. 404.

[f] Williams, T. A. Some Plants Injurious to Stock. S. Dak. Agric. Coll. and Exper. Sta. Bul. 33, p. 21. 1893.

[g] Givens, A. J. Loco or Crazy Weed. Med. Century, vol. 1, p. 22. 1893.

[h] Eastwood, A., l. c. 1892.

[i] Sayre, L. E. Loco Weed. Amer. Vet. Rev., vol. 11, p. 555. 1887.

[j] Amer. Pharm. Assoc. Proc. for 1879, vol. 27, p. 611. 1880.

[k] Kelsey, F. D. Another Loco Plant. Bot. Gaz., vol. 14, p. 20. 1889.

[l] Sayre, L. E. Loco Weed. Kans. State Board Agric., 5th Bienn. Rept., p. 209. 1887.

[m] Anderson, F. W. Poisonous Plants and the Symptoms They Produce. Bot. Gaz., vol. 14, p. 180. 1889.—Pammel, L. H. Loco Weeds. Vis Medicatrix, vol. 1, p. 44. 1891.

showing more or less stupor it is said to be locoed.[a] The early Spanish settlers seemed to be unfamiliar with the disease, or at least of any causative relation between the plant and the disease. The Spanish name for *Astragalus mollissimus* was " Garbanzillo," from its resemblance to Garbanzo (*Cicer arietinum*), which is used in Spain as a food.[b] The term as applied to this condition seems to be of comparatively recent origin.[c]

A somewhat similar condition to the loco in stock is sometimes attributed by the ranchmen of our Western States to eating various sages.[d] In Texas the loco disease is known as " grass staggers."[e]

Hayes [f] has described as follows a condition known as grass staggers, which apparently has little resemblance to loco and is supposed to be due to eating overripe grass, especially rye.

The symptoms, generally, take two or three days to become developed. The animal gradually becomes more or less unconscious and paralyzed and staggers if forced to walk. Although he may have great difficulty in keeping on his legs, he is extremely averse from going down and leans for support against any convenient object. He breathes in a snoring manner. The mucous membranes are tinged with yellow. Convulsions, or spasms, like those of tetanus, may come on.

Recovery may be expected in cases which are not marked by extreme symptoms.

If animals are not regularly salted, they visit salt deposits and eat the alkalis. This some sheepmen believe to be the cause of the locoed condition, but this is disproved by the occurrence of locoed animals in ranges without salt. Others modify this view by claiming that the vitiation in taste from eating these alkalis leads to a desire for the loco weeds and thus to the locoed condition.[g]

---

[a] Stalker, M. The " Loco " Plant and Its Effect on Animals. Bur. Animal Industry, 3d Ann. Rept. (1886), p. 275. 1887.—Anderson, F. W. Poisonous Plants and the Symptoms They Produce. Bot. Gaz., vol. 14, p. 180. 1889.

NOTE.—The symptoms described in Janvier's interesting story, "In Old Mexico " (Scribner's Magazine, vol. 1, p. 67, 1887), would coincide with those due to some member of the nightshade family (probably *Datura stramonium*). See also Pilgrim, C. W., Does the Loco Weed Produce Insanity? in Proc. Amer. Medico-Psycholog. Assoc., vol. 5, p. 167. 1898.

[b] Sayre, L. E. Loco Weed. Kans. State Board Agric., 5th Bienn. Rept., p. 209. 1887.

[c] Stalker, M. The " Loco " Plant and Its Effect on Animals. Bur. Animal Industry, 3d Ann. Rept. (1886), p. 272. 1887.

[d] Mayo, N. S. Loco. The Industrialist, vol. 30, p. 473. 1904.

[e] Science, vol. 9, p. 32. 1887.

[f] Hayes, M. H. Veterinary Notes for Horse Owners, London, 1903, p. 425.—Compare Woronin, M. Ueber die Taumelgetreide in Süd-Ussurien. Bot. Zeit., vol. 49, p. 80. 1891.

[g] Chesnut, V. K., and Wilcox, E. V. Stock-Poisoning Plants of Montana. U. S. Dept. Agric., Div. Bot., Bul. 26, p. 88. 1901.

NOTE.—The wide distribution of these plants is claimed to be partly due to the buffalo. See Blankinship, J. W., The Loco and Some Other Poisonous Plants in Montana, in Mont. Agric. Exper. Sta. Bul. 45, p. 79. 1903.

CLINICAL SYMPTOMS OF LOCOED ANIMALS AS DESCRIBED IN LITERATURE.

The animals usually affected are sheep, horses, cattle, mules,[a] donkeys,[b] and goats. It is claimed that practically all herbivorous animals are liable to the disease, even antelopes being affected.[c] Hogs are said to be unaffected,[d] but definite information is lacking. Cows seem to be less sensitive to this form of intoxication.[e] The condition is usually a chronic one, although acute cases are said to occur at times. The symptoms consist of digestive disturbances, associated with emaciation and various symptoms suggesting lesions in the nervous system, central or peripheral. The animals lose their appetite from the first, begin to emaciate, and show symptoms of malnutrition and starvation. The head trembles, the gait becomes feeble and uncertain, the eyes become sunken and have a " flat, glassy look."[f] There is a general sluggishness, muscular incoordination, and difficulty in motion; finally all control of the limbs is lost and the animal is unable to stand; the coat becomes rough and loses its luster, and, in fact, all the typical symptoms of starvation appear. In some cases diarrhea is also present.

All of Nockolds's animals, however, were constipated and the stools were covered with mucus.[g] The dependent portions of the body may swell, simply as an expression of the anæmia.[h] Sometimes there are symptoms indicating acute pain,[i] the animals running about as if affected with colic. They may belch and their abdomens swell. Some claim that the animals are markedly salivated so that the saliva trickles from their mouths. In other cases the mouth may be dry.[j] The eyes may be rolled up so that the whites alone show. In some cases the pupil has been noted to be dilated, as in atropine

---

[a] Kingsley, B. F. The Loco Plant. Daniel's Texas Medical Journal, vol. 3, p. 522. 1888.

[b] Schwartzkopff, O. The Effects of " Loco-Weed." Amer. Vet. Rev., vol. 12, p. 162. 1888.

[c] McCullaugh, F. A. Locoed Horses. Journ. Comp. Med. & Vet. Archives, vol. 13, p. 435. 1892.

[d] Eastwood, A. The Loco Weeds. Zoe, vol. 3, p. 57. 1892.

[e] Vasey, G. Plants Poisonous to Cattle in California. Report of Commissioner of Agriculture for 1874, p. 159. 1875.

[f] Vasey, G., l. c., p. 159.

[g] Nockolds, C. Poisoning by Loco Weed. Amer. Vet. Rev., vol. 20, p. 570. 1896–7.

[h] Patterson, A. H. Starvation Œdema. Med. Rev., vol. 56, p. 715, 1899.

[i] Vasey, G. Botanical Notes, Monthly Reports of Dept. Agriculture for 1873, p. 504. 1874.

[j] Anderson, F. W. Poisonous Plants and the Symptoms They Produce. Bot. Gaz., vol. 14, p. 180. 1889.

poisoning,[a] but Wilcox states that they are contracted as after the use of eserine.[b] The temperature of the animal falls from $\frac{1}{2}$ degree to $1\frac{1}{2}$ degrees F. below normal.[c] Tetanic symptoms may occur,[d] or the muscles of the mouth and tongue becoming paralyzed may interfere with mastication. When water is offered to the animal, it gazes stupidly at it and may not drink for days. One of the symptoms noted is the loss of power to back properly.[e] Cows during the first two or three months of gestation are almost sure to abort.[f] This is claimed by Knowles, however, to be due to malnutrition. As a result of these observations, suggesting some uterine action, the drug has been proposed as an emmenagogue.[g]

The psychical symptoms are shown by errors of judgment. The animal becomes dull and spiritless and wanders about half dazed. The mental dullness passes into stupor. This dull, stupid condition has been compared to intoxication with opium. If the locoed horse is led across a stick lying on the ground he often jumps high as if it were a great obstacle. The animal may now have maniacal attacks, during which he rears and may fall backward,[h] and makes unreasonable jumps and other unexpected movements, thus rendering himself dangerous to man.[i] Other symptoms due to disturbances of the central nervous system are hallucinations of various sorts. Though the optic nerve itself is apparently not affected, the animal will stare at an object for a long time without any apparent comprehension of its nature. This disturbance in the visual function McCullaugh claims to be one of the first symptoms of this disease. The animal seems to lose all idea of distance, as he will butt against an obstruction as if oblivious of its presence. Any sudden or violent motion made before him may cause him to fall. According to some,

---

[a] Schwartzkopff, O. The Effects of "Loco-Weed." Amer. Vet. Rev., vol. 12, p. 161. 1888.

[b] Wilcox, T. E. Treatment of "Loco" Poisoning in Idaho Territory. Med. Rec., vol. 31, p. 268. 1887.

[c] Mayo, N. S. Some Observations Upon Loco. Kans. State Agric. Coll. Bul. 35, p. 118. 1893.

[d] McCullaugh, F. A. Locoed Horses. Journ. Comp. Med. and Vet. Archives, vol. 13, p. 436. 1892.

[e] O'Brine, D. Progress Bulletin on the Loco and Larkspur. Colo. State Agric. Coll. Bul. 25, p. 12. 1893.

[f] Knowles, M. E. Loco Poisoning. Breeders' Gaz., vol. 39, p. 973. 1901.— Sayre, L. E. Loco Weed. Kans. State Board of Agric., 5th Bienn. Rept., p. 211. 1887.—Ruedi, C. Loco Weed. Trans. Colo. State Med. Soc., p. 422. 1895.

[g] Miller, C. H. The Loco Weed: Its Probable Usefulness as an Emmenagogue. Southern Clinic, vol. 11, p. 269. 1888.

[h] Vasey, G. Botanical Notes. Monthly Reports of Dept. Agriculture for 1873, p. 504. 1874.

[i] Parker, W. T. The Loco-Weed. Science, vol. 23, p. 101. 1894.

the animal loses the sense which guides him in finding water. A cow may fail to recognize her calf.[a] There is more or less loss of control of the limbs [b] and tremors;[c] the feet are lifted abnormally high when trotting, and, if crowded, the animal falls headlong and will jump over little hollows as if they were wide ditches.[d] The horse may shy without apparent cause and kick at imaginary objects,[e] and, in fact, the reasoning powers seem to be lost. These attacks are brought on by sudden excitement or when crossing water.[f] There may be cutaneous hyperæsthesia.

The animals may remain with the herd, but they often wander away. Stalker records the following observations:

> I have seen a single animal miles away from any other individual of the herd, carefully searching as if for some lost object, and when a loco plant is found he would devour every morsel of it with the greatest relish. As soon as one plant was eaten he would immediately go in search of more, apparently oblivious to everything but the intoxication afforded by his one favorite article of food.[g]

All of Nockolds's animals which were locoed were mares more than 6 years of age.[h]

According to Stalker there is a passive type in which the animal shows symptoms only on being disturbed; the animal then becomes unmanageable. This happens even with old, well-broken saddle horses.[i]

There are few published reports as to the symptoms occurring in sheep which are locoed. Stalker [j] says sheep " become loco-eaters, grow stupid, emaciated, and eventually die." One of the few descriptions of the symptoms is that of Ruedi,[k] in which he claims that

---

[a] Vasey, G. Botanical Notes. Monthly Reports of Dept. Agriculture for 1874, p. 513. 1875.

[b] Anderson, F. W. Poisonous Plants and the Symptoms They Produce. Bot. Gaz., vol. 14, p. 180. 1889.

[c] Sayre, L. E. Loco Weed. Proc. Amer. Pharm. Assoc., vol. 36, p. 111. 1888.

[d] Nockolds, C. Poisoning by Loco Weed. Amer. Vet. Rev., vol. 20, p. 570. 1896–7.

[e] Knowles, M. E. Loco Poisoning. Breeders' Gaz., vol. 39, p. 972. 1901.

[f] Vasey, G. Botanical Notes. Monthly Reports of Dept. Agriculture for 1873, p. 504. 1874.

[g] Stalker, M. The "Loco" Plant and Its Effect on Animals. Bur. Animal Industry, 3d Ann. Rept. (1886), p. 272. 1887.—Nockolds, C. Poisoning by Loco Weed. Amer. Vet. Rev., vol. 20, p. 570. 1896–7.—Maisch, J. M. Poisonous Species of Astragalus. Amer. Journ. Pharm., vol. 51, p. 239. 1879.

[h] Nockolds, C. Poisoning by Loco Weed. Amer. Vet. Rev., vol. 20, p. 570. 1896–7.

[i] Stalker, M., l. c., p. 273.

[j] Stalker, M., l. c., p. 274.

[k] Ruedi, C. Loco Weed (Astragalus Mollissimus) : A Toxico-Chemical Study. Trans. Colo. State Med. Soc., 1895, p. 417.

the symptoms in sheep are those comparable to the symptoms of cerebro-spinal meningitis except that there is an absence of fever. Ruedi speaks of sheep " lying flat on the ground, not able to stand, and not able even to lift their heads to drink the offered water; the head and the vertebra in opisthotonus position; the four legs stretched out and stiff; breathing was stertorous, pulse slow, abdomen much distended, diarrhea present. * * * The heart * * * was very slow and insufficient." The teeth (in sheep) may blacken and fall out.[a]

It is mainly the young animals, such as lambs and colts, that are affected, probably due to the fact that their attention is more easily directed to the flower of the loco [b] plants. It is claimed (on slight evidence) that men have become locoed. The symptoms in them are nausea and headache.[c]

Schuchardt [d] has called attention to the resemblance of the symptoms in locoed animals to those which occur in so-called lathyrism, but most observers in this country have especially marked the resemblance of the symptoms to those induced by the habitual use of narcotic drugs.[e]

As a rule the loco plants are refused by animals save when there is lack of other food, although at times animals have shown the keenest relish for these plants, rejected all other forage, and devoted their whole attention to searching for the loco plants.[f]

Stalker says that animals not too long addicted to the use of these plants, if confined, soon lose their taste for them (after two or three months),[g] although old loco eaters do not readily lose the habit. Stalker also says that " it is to be presumed that the plant is possessed

---

[a] Blankinship, J. W. Loco and Some Other Poisonous Plants in Montana. Mont. Agric. Exper. Sta. Bul. 45, p. 81. 1903.

[b] Blankinship, J. W., l. c.

[c] Day, M. G. Loco-Weed. In F. P. Foster's Reference Book of Practical Therapeutics, vol. 1, p. 588. 1896.—Pilgrim, C. W. Does the Loco-Weed Produce Insanity? Proc. Amer. Medico-Psycholog. Assoc., vol. 5, p. 167. 1898.

[d] Schuchardt, B. Die Loco-Krankheit der Pferde und des Rindviehs. Deutsch. Zeits. f. Thiermed., vol. 18, p. 405. 1892.—Parker, W. T. Loco-Weed. Science, vol. 23, p. 101. 1894.

[e] McCullaugh, F. A. Locoed Horses. Journ. Comp. Med. and Vet. Archives, vol. 13, p. 435. 1892.

[f] Stalker, M. The "Loco" Plant and Its Effect on Animals. Bur. Animal Industry, 3d Ann. Rept. (1886), p. 272. 1887.

[g] Stalker, M. The "Loco" Plant and Its Effect on Animals. Bur. Animal Industry, 3d Ann. Rept. (1886), p. 272. 1887.—See also Linfield, F. B. Sheep Feeding, in Mont. Agric. Coll. Exper. Sta. Bul., 59. 1905.—Special Report on Diseases of Cattle. Bur. Animal Industry, 1904, p. 66.—Wilcox, E. V. Plant Poisoning of Stock in Montana. Bur. Animal Industry, 17th Ann. Rept., p. 115. 1900.

of some toxic property that has a specific effect on the nervous centers, and that these effects have a marked tendency to remain permanent." [a]

The fundamental character of the disorder seems to be a progressing anæmia. The interpretation of psychical symptoms in herbivora, and especially on the range, must often be fallacious.

CONDITIONS SIMILAR TO LOCO-WEED POISONING IN OTHER PARTS OF THE WORLD.

According to Maiden [b] a condition similar to loco is met with among animals in Australia and is there believed to be due to eating various species of Swainsona. [c] As Maiden says, " Its effect on sheep is well known; they separate from the flock, wander about listlessly, and are known to the shepherds as ' pea-eaters ' or ' indigo-eaters.' When once a sheep takes to eating this plant it seldom or never fattens, and may be said to be lost to its owner." Horses, after eating this herb, " were exceptionally difficult to catch, and it was observed how strange they appeared. Their eyes were staring out of their heads and they were prancing against trees and stumps. The second day two out of nine died, and five others had to be left at the camp."

Martin [d] experimentally studied these cases of intoxication and sums up his work as follows:

1. That one can by feeding sheep upon Darling pea reproduce all the symptoms which are attributed by pastoralists to this cause. Briefly stated these symptoms are: Stupidity, loss of alertness and an agonized expression, followed by stiffness and slight staggering and frequently trembling of the head or limbs. Later, clumsiness and unsteadiness ensue, which slowly advance until the animal often falls down. In this stage, the action of the animal in running over small obstacles is characteristic. It jumps over a twig as if it were a foot in height. When first it commences to tumble about, it is able more or less readily to regain its feet, but in the advanced stage of the disease this is impossible and, after exhausting itself in efforts to do so, it remains lying down until it dies. During the whole time the sheep become progressively more bloodless, and in advanced cases the blood when shed appears to the naked eye lighter in color. It contains fewer red blood-cells (about two-thirds to one-half the usual number). (The corpuscles were estimated in several cases by means of a hæmocytometer.) All these symptoms are much aggravated by driving. Thus, an animal in which the symptoms are little marked may exhibit them in a striking degree after being driven. In addition to the above the teeth

---

[a] Stalker, M., l. c., p. 275.

[b] Maiden, J. H. Plants Reputed to be Poisonous to Stock in Australia. Dept. Agric., New South Wales, Misc. Pub. No. 477, pp. 15, 16. 1901.

[c] Notes on Some American and Australian Plants Injurious to Stock. Agric. Gaz., New South Wales, vol. 4, p. 677. 1894.—Notes on Weeds. The Darling Pea. Agric. Gaz., New South Wales, vol. 3, p. 330. 1893.

[d] Martin, C. J. Report on an Investigation into the Effects of Darling Pea (Swainsona Galegifolia) upon Sheep. Agric. Gaz., New South Wales, vol. 8, p. 366. 1898.

(especially in young sheep) frequently become loose, and consequently displaced or even dislodged.

2. That the time which elapses before the onset of definite symptoms is three to four weeks in sheep of 2 to 3 years old. (It is probable, however, that with younger animals the time is shorter.)

3. That under the conditions of the experiment, the animals survived about three months. They lived, however, an invalid's life. Everything was brought to them, and it is improbable that if feeding exclusively upon the pea, and left to shift for themselves in the paddocks, they would survive more than two months.

4. That if a sheep be returned to proper fodder after one month to six weeks feeding upon the pea, and before the symptoms are fully established, it may recover completely.

5. That when once the paralytic symptoms are established it will not recover; but if returned to proper food, will remain in much the same condition, becoming neither better nor worse.

6. That Darling pea contains a very fair amount of nourishing material so that animals may, provided they eat it readily, retain their condition on it for some weeks, until the poisonous principle contained has had time to exert its effects.

These plants, if fed with other herbage, do not seem to be injurious and apparently lose their harmful action upon being cultivated.[a] As long as salt is properly fed the animals will not eat this plant[b] and are said to suffer no effects from it. Physiological study has shown the presence of a body with marked sudorific power which causes rapid emaciation in frogs.[c]

It has been claimed that these symptoms are due to the presence of a narcotic poison in the plant.[d] Post-mortem examinations were negative save for the presence of a peripheral neuritis.[e]

---

[a] Woolls, W. On the Forage-Plants Indigenous in New South Wales. Linn. Soc., New South Wales, Proc., vol. 7, pp. 315–316. 1882.

[b] Guthrie, F. B., and Turner, F. Supposed Poisonous Plant. Agric. Gaz., New South Wales, vol. 4, p. 86. 1894.

[c] Bailey, F. M., and Gordon, P. R. Plants Reputed Poisonous and Injurious to Stock, Brisbane, 1887, p. 25.

[d] Guthrie, F. B., and Turner, F. Supposed Poisonous Plant. Agric. Gaz., New South Wales, vol. 4, p. 87. 1894·

[e] Martin, C. J. Report on the Investigation into the Effects of Darling Pea (Swainsona Galegifolia) upon Sheep. Agric. Gaz., New South Wales, vol. 8, p. 367. 1898. (Further literature on the indigo disease will be found in Bailey, F. M., and Gordon, P. R. Plants Reputed Poisonous and Injurious to Stock, Brisbane, 1887, p. 25).

NOTE.—In Canada a chronic disease associated with cirrhosis of the liver results from eating ragwort, or *Senecio jacobaea*. See Dept. of Agriculture, Canada, Rept. of Veterinary Director General, 1905, Ottawa, 1906, p. 31.—In South Africa a disorder known as nenta appears in goats after eating certain plants, especially *Cotyledon ventricosa*. See Hutcheon, D., Nenta, in Agric. Journ. Cape of Good Hope, vol. 14, p. 862. 1899.

PATHOLOGICAL CONDITIONS IN LOCOED ANIMALS AS DESCRIBED ON THE RANGE.

The pathological features as described by previous writers are a softening and ulceration of the stomach walls [a] and a degeneration of the walls of the intestines with or without perforations. The peritoneum may be found inflamed.[b] The peritoneum and omentum in one case (cow), reported by Sayre, were covered with small nodules. These were probably tubercular in origin. The colon in one horse was found enormously distended, while the cœcum and small intestines were normal,[c] save that the walls appeared thin.

Ulcers have been found at times in the kidneys, but were probably secondary in origin, as other cases are reported with normal kidneys. Faville has found in some cases amyloid degeneration. The pancreas and spleen are reported normal. The abdominal cavity may contain a slight effusion.[d] The liver has been found cirrhotic, and at times shows tubercular lesions of a secondary nature. The inner coat of the bladder has been found softened, and in sheep the bladder may be markedly distended at the autopsy. The cerebral membranes are congested and perhaps adherent,[e] and there may be blood clots over the longitudinal sinus or at the base of the brain. Effusions have been especially noted around the medulla. The arachnoid has also shown slight congestion, and in other cases the membranes showed a slight thickening. The middle ventricle was found filled with yellow serum, while the fourth ventricle contained a hemorrhagic effusion,[f] and the base of the brain was covered by a clot. The hemorrhage may become organized and the brain be held to the membranes by tough organized fibers. In many cases serous effusion is present in the lateral ventricles. The arachnoid space is also in some cases similarly filled. Microscopic examination of the brain in the case of a steer showed atrophy of Purkinjie's cells.[g]

In sheep the post-mortem examination showed paleness, anæmia of the muscles, and great distention of the abdomen. The intestines

---

[a] Anderson, F. W. Poisonous Plants and the Symptoms They Produce. Bot. Gaz., vol. 14, p. 180. 1889.

[b] Sayre, L. E. Loco Weed. Amer. Vet. Rev., vol. 11, p. 558. 1887.

[c] O'Brine, D. Progress Bulletin on the Loco and Larkspur. Colo. State Agric. Coll. Bul. 25, p. 12. 1893.

[d] Faville, in O'Brine, D. Progress Bulletin on the Loco and Larkspur. Colo. State Agric. Coll. Bul. 25, p. 11. 1893.

[e] Sayre, L. E. Loco Weed. Amer. Vet. Rev., vol. 11, p. 559. 1887.

[f] Stalker, M. The "Loco" Plant and Its Effect on Animals. Bur. Animal Industry, 3d Ann. Rept. (1886), p. 274. 1887.—Sayre, L. E. Loco-Weed. Amer. Pharm. Assoc. Proc., vol. 38, p. 108. 1890.—O'Brine, D. Progress Bulletin on the Loco and Larkspur. Colo. State Agric. Coll. Bul. 25, pp. 16, 17. 1893.

[g] Mayo, N. S., l. c., p. 118.

were found filled with gases, and the mesenteric blood vessels filled with blood. No peritonitis, or ascites, or ecchymoses in the mucous membranes were noted in the autopsies made on sheep by Ruedi. The liver has been seen enlarged. In sheep the brain was anæmic. Microscopically the brain showed atrophy and the Purkinjie's cells disappeared or their processes atrophied. In these sheep the brain was so anæmic that the distinction between the gray and the white matter was hard to define.[a] The membranes of the cord have been found inflamed and adherent, but the spinal cord was usually normal.[b] In some cases, however, the spinal cord has been found softened [c] and œdematous. The arteries of the limbs were gorged with blood,[d] and at the same time there was a collection of serum in the abdominal cavity. ·Death is thought to be due to starvation.[e] In other words, the pathological condition, according to published accounts, shows little that is characteristic save some action on the gastro-intestinal tract.

HISTORICAL SKETCH OF LOCO INVESTIGATIONS FROM A PHARMACOLOGICAL STANDPOINT.

During the western immigration of 1849 the Indians along the Missouri River described to the immigrants a plant (*Astragalus mollissimus*) producing death in horses and cattle, which was preceded by various forms of excitement.[f]

The attention of the United States Department of Agriculture was first called to the toxic action of the loco plants in 1873, when specimens of the plants, which were identified as *Astragalus hornii* and *A. lentiginosus*,[g] were sent from California by Mr. O. B. Ormsby, with

[a] Ruedi, C. Loco Weed (Astragalus Mollissimus) : A Toxico-Chemical Study. Trans. Colo. State Med. Soc., 1895, p. 418.

[b] Sayre, L. E. Loco Weed. Amer. Vet. Rev., vol. 11, p. 559. 1887.

[c] O'Brine, D. Progress Bulletin on the Loco and Larkspur. Colo. State Agric. Coll. Bul. 25, p. 12. 1893.—Klench, J. P. Rattleweed or Loco Disease. Amer. Vet. Rev., vol 12, p. 399. 1888.

[d] Anderson, F. W. Poisonous Plants and the Symptoms They Produce. Bot. Gaz., vol. 14, p. 180. 1889.

[e] McCullaugh, F. A. Locoed Horses. Journ. Comp. Med. and Vet. Archives, vol. 13, p. 436. 1892.

[f] Storke, B. F. The Loco Weed. Med. Current, vol. 8, p. 155. 1892.—Kellogg, A. California and Colorado " Loco " Poisons. Cal. Acad. Sci. Proc. for 1875, vol. 6, p. 3. ˙1876˙

NOTE.—The very early reports of these loco plants were purely botanical. See Torrey, J., Botany, in Report on the United States and Mexican Boundary Survey, by W. H. Emory, vol. 2, p. 56, 1859; also Botanical Register, London, vol. 13, pl. 1054, 1827.

[g] Vasey, G. Plants Poisonous to Cattle in· California. Rept. of Commissioner of Agriculture for 1874, p. 159. 1875.

the statement that they were poisonous to stock, especially to horses. Mrs. J. S. Whipple also corroborated this information. The botanist of the Department, Dr. George Vasey,[a] published a note and requested further information concerning the plants. These notes were enlarged by a similar contribution by Dr. P. Moffat on *Aragallus lamberti.*[b] The following year Vasey reported with more fullness, and his description of the action of the plants is substantially what we find in most of the books of to-day.

In 1876 Lemmon[c] noted that *Astragalus mortoni* was "a deadly sheep poison." At the same time Rothrock,[d] botanist of the United States Geographical Survey under Lieutenant Wheeler, described these plants, and Kellogg,[e] a botanist in California, reported that *Astragalus menziesii* was causing great losses in horses, sheep, and cattle and claimed that the stockmen had been familiar with this disorder for at least ten or fifteen years. This report of Kellogg was followed by that of Rothrock[f] in 1877.

In 1876 a specimen of *Aragallus lamberti* was sent from Colorado to Professor Prescott, of the University of Michigan, under the name of "crazy weed," with the statement that it was poisonous to horses and cattle and that, while the Mexicans often used it in making beer, it sometimes caused symptoms in men. His pupil, Miss Watson, undertook a study of its chemical properties. She failed to isolate any pure chemical compound, but claimed that in the root there was a body giving alkaloidal reactions and that there was also a resinous body present. Another of his pupils, W. R. Birdsall, took the ground-up root himself in doses of 20 grains at various intervals for several days and later 40-grain doses in one and a half hours, but without experiencing any marked symptoms except colicky pains. A kitten also was given about one and a half ounces of the fluid extract without effect. Prescott[g] sums up by saying that "it would seem that the dried ground root possesses no poisonous properties." The work of Miss Watson was considered of sufficient importance to be abstracted

---

[a] Vasey, G. Botanical Notes. Monthly Reports of Dept. Agriculture for 1873, p. 503. 1874.

[b] Vasey, G. Botanical Notes. Monthly Reports of Dept. Agriculture for 1874, p. 513. 1875.

[c] Brewer, W. H., and Watson, S. Geological Survey of California, Botany, vol. 1, p. 155. 1876.

[d] Rothrock, J. T. Notes on Economic Botany, in G. M. Wheeler's Report upon U. S. Geographical Surveys West of the One Hundredth Meridian, vol. 6, p. 43. 1878.

[e] Kellogg, A. California and Colorado Loco Poisons. Cal. Academy of Sciences, Proc., 1875, vol. 6, p. 3. 1876.

[f] Rothrock, J. T. Poisonous Properties of the Leguminosæ. Acad. of Nat. Sci., Phila., Proc., vol. 29, p. 274. 1877.

[g] Prescott, A. B. Laboratory Notes—A Partial Analysis of the Oxytropis Lamberti. Amer. Journ. Pharm., vol. 50, p. 564. 1878.

in the Annual Report of the Commissioner of Agriculture for 1878 (1879), page 134.

Gradually the Department of Agriculture became more and more interested in this subject, and Peter Collier, chief chemist, in 1878, examined the roots and leaves of *Aragallus lamberti* for alkaloids, but found none.[a]

In 1880 Peter Collier published a proximate analysis of *Astragalus mollissimus* made by Francis A. Wentz, of Kansas. His investigations showed it to have an ash content of 6.76 per cent, while the *Aragallus lamberti*, analyzed by L. F. Dyrenforth, of Chicago, showed an ash content of 4.32 per cent. Collier[b] sums up by saying:

From the additional work done at this Department it seems probable that the deleterious effects observed from animals eating this plant may be due principally to the fact that the sweet taste causes cattle to reject more nutritious food and strive to subsist upon the Oxytropis only. This plant is mechanically a very unfit substance for food, being of a tough, fibrous, and indigestible character. It is possible that, when the animal becomes somewhat enfeebled by lack of proper nourishment, the small amount of alkaloid may have a direct poisonous action. Again, it seems probable that the plant may contain much larger proportions of alkaloid at certain stages in its development than at others, or the seeds may prove to be the most injurious portion.

The departmental work was continued by further short notices by Vasey[c] in 1884, 1886, and 1887, and by the report of Stalker in 1887. This report by Stalker is still the best description on the clinical side of the question.

Rothrock,[d] meeting the loco plants in his survey work, describes their effects on animals as follows:

Certain it is, however, that, once commenced, they continue it, passing through temporary intoxication to a complete nervous and muscular wreck in the later stages, when it has developed into a fully marked disease which terminates in death from starvation or inability to digest a more nourishing food. The animal toward the last becomes stupid or wild, or even vicious, or, again, acting as though attacked with "blind staggers."

Under the name of Crotalaria, H. Gibbons,[e] in 1879, refers to a plant growing in California which it was claimed was producing characteristic symptoms of poisoning in horses and sheep. This plant Professor Maisch afterwards identified as *Aragallus lamberti*.

---

[a] Rept. of Commissioner of Agriculture for 1878, p. 134. 1879.

[b] Rept. of Commissioner of Agriculture for 1879, pp. 89, 90. 1880.

[c] Rept. of Commissioner of Agriculture for 1886, p. 75. 1887. Rept. of Commissioner of Agriculture for 1884, p. 123. 1884.

[d] Rothrock, J. T. Notes on Economic Botany, in G. M. Wheeler's Report upon U. S. Geographical Surveys West of the One Hundredth Meridian, vol. 6, p. 43. 1878.

[e] Gibbons, H. Poisonous Effects of Crotallaria—Vulgo Rattle Weed, Loco Weed. Pacific Med. and Surg. Journ., vol. 21, p. 496. 1878–79.

Dr. Isaac Ott[a] undertook the physiological study of the question and used an alcoholic extract of *Astragalus mollissimus*. He found from its action on frogs, rabbits, and cats that the plant had decided physiological action, as follows:

(1) It decreases the irritability of the motor nerves.

(2) Greatly affects the sensory ganglia of the central nervous system, preventing them from readily receiving impressions.

(3) Has a spinal tetanic action.

(4) Kills mainly by arrest of the heart.

(5) Increases the salivary secretion.

(6) Has a stupefying action on the brain.

(7) Reduces the cardiac force and frequency.

(8) Temporarily increases arterial tension, but finally decreases it.

(9) It greatly dilates the pupil.

Doctor Stockman, in England, about this time tried the action of the aqueous and alcoholic extracts of the dried *Astragalus mollissimus* sent from Texas. He experimented with frogs and rabbits in increasing doses, but without result.[b]

In 1888 Hill reported that a species of Astragalus was acting detrimentally on cattle, goats, and sheep in Cyprus and that these animals fell down as if intoxicated, and also that the natives·in time of great drought feed their cattle with this plant mixed with straw, but that they were always made sick until they became used to it.

In 1885 Professor Sayre, of the University of Kansas, undertook the investigation of the loco question. His first report was made in the Transactions of the Kansas Academy of Sciences for 1885, and his reports have been continued at various periods up to 1904. The results of his experiments on various animals—dogs, cats, and frogs[c]—have been entirely negative. He administered alcoholic preparations to himself and took them until they became too nauseous to continue, and found they produced absolutely no symptoms besides the nausea. He suggests, however, that if the plant really is poisonous it is due to its fine hairs, which might mechanically cause death. Sayre has stated that he has sent thousands of pounds of the dried loco plants to various investigators in America and Europe, but all reports were negative as to pharmacological activity. He has, however, done some work on the pure chemistry of the plant and found that the plant contained 10 per cent of moisture and yielded 12.01 per cent of ash. Of this ash, 25 per cent was soluble in water, while 50.6 per cent was soluble in HCl. The insoluble portion consisted

---

[a] Ott, I. Physiological Action of Astragalus Mollissimus. New Remedies, vol. 11, p. 227. 1882.

[b] Hill, J. R. Note on a Species of Astragalus from Cyprus. Pharm. Journ. and Trans., 3 s., vol. 18, p. 712. 1887–88.

[c] Sayre, L. E. Loco-Weed. Proc. Amer. Pharm. Assoc., vol. 36, p. 112. 1888.

largely of silica. He found CaO, K_2O, MgO, Al_2O_3, and Fe_2O_3, with the acid radicals SO_3, Cl, P_2O_5, CO_2, and SiO_2.[a] Although Sayre claims that the plant is physiologically inactive, he tried by chemical means to isolate a physiologically active body and, naturally enough under the circumstances, failed to find one. He claims that while the plant might give alkaloid reactions, he was unable to isolate this body in a pure state, and that alfalfa reacted similarly.

The investigation on animals was continued by Kennedy.[b] He administered an infusion of ½ ounce of green *Astragalus mollissimus* to a fasting dog weighing .23 pounds, but there were no symptoms after 12 hours. A decoction of 1 ounce of the green plant and one of 4 ounces of the dried plant were likewise without action. Extracts with hydrochloric acid were also inactive. When 400 grams of the dried and powdered plant were fed in substance the result was merely to increase the appetite. The organic acid obtained from 4 ounces of the plant was also found to be inert.

Kennedy did not state in what season the plant was collected and from what locality it was obtained, but says simply that the plant extract was inactive to a dog, a carnivorous animal, and that therefore the plant is nonpoisonous. He adds that death might be due to the tough fibers and indigestible character of the plant. He overlooks, however, the fact that the plant might vary in its toxicity, and he infers from the experiments on carnivorous animals that these results would hold good for herbivora, yet he does not claim that carnivora become locoed in nature.

Kennedy found that the plant lost 80 per cent in weight on drying and that the water extract which represented 30.6 per cent of the powdered and dried plant contained magnesium sulphate and sodium chlorid, tannic acid, gum, coloring matter, an extractive, and a " peculiar organic acid." The ashed plant yielded 20 per cent of ash, consisting of magnesium sulphate, sodium chlorid, alumina, silica, and a trace of iron. " The abundant precipitate produced by the alkaline hydrates, potassium, sodium, and ammonium was found to consist of magnesium hydrate, an abundance of this base being present in the plant." Kennedy also obtained alkaloidal reactions, but failed to isolate the body giving these reactions.

In 1889 the investigations were greatly stimulated by the report of Doctor Day,[c] then of the University of Michigan. She claimed that she was able to produce marked physiological symptoms, using both *Astragalus mollissimus* and *Aragallus lamberti* in her work. She

---

[a] Sayre, L. E. Loco Weed. Amer. Vet. Rev., vol. 11, p. 556. 1887.

[b] Kennedy, J. Loco Weed (Crazy Weed). Pharm. Rec., vol. 8, p. 197. 1888.

[c] Day, M. G. Experimental Demonstrations of the Toxicity of the " Loco Weed." N. Y. Med. Journ., vol. 49, p. 237. 1889.

administered daily 60 to 70 c. c. of a decoction [a] of the plants to kittens, together with abundant milk and other food. She states that in two days—

The kittens became less active, the coat grew rough, appetite for ordinary food diminished and fondness for the "loco" increased, diarrhea came on, and retching and vomiting occasionally occurred. The expression became peculiar and characteristic. Emaciation and the above symptoms progressively increased until the eighteenth day, when periods of convulsive excitement supervened. At times the convulsions were tetanic in character; frothing at the mouth and throwing the head backward as in opisthotonus were marked. At other times the kitten would stand on its hind legs and strike the air with its forepaws, then fall backward and throw itself from side to side. These periods of excitement were followed by perfect quiet, the only apparent sign of life being the respiratory movements. After a short interval of quiet the convulsive movements would recur. These alternate periods of excitement and quiet lasted thirty-six hours, when the posterior extremities became paralyzed, and the kitten died about two hours afterward. There was no apparent loss of consciousness before death.

The post-mortem examination revealed the presence of ulcers in the stomach and duodenum. Some of the ulcers had nearly perforated the walls of the stomach and duodenum. The heart was in diastole; brain and myel appeared normal. As might be expected from the emaciated condition, the entire body was anæmic.

In a second case 60 to 70 cubic centimeters of a more concentrated decoction were fed daily, with other food as before, to a vigorous adult cat. The symptoms of inactivity, loss of appetite, rough coat, diarrhea, and the peculiar expression of countenance were as in the first case. By the twelfth day the cat was wasted almost to a skeleton, and was correspondingly weak. Paralysis of the hind limbs came on, and the cat died on the thirteenth day. There were no periods of excitement in this case.

These cats developed a craving for the decoction and " would beg for it as an ordinary kitten does for milk, and when supplied would lie down contented."

Doctor Day made controls with healthy animals under the same conditions, with the exception that they received no loco plant. She also fed a young wild jack rabbit on milk and grass for a few days and then substituted fresh loco plants for grass.

At first the "loco" was refused, but after two or three days the "loco" was eaten with as much relish as the grass had been. After ten days of the milk and "loco" diet the rabbit was found dead, with the head thrown back and the stomach ruptured.

Subcutaneous injections of the concentrated decoction caused nervous twitchings in frogs and kittens, and if large amounts were used death followed in from one to two hours from paralysis of the heart. The same symptoms were produced in frogs by the injection of an alcoholic extract of the residue left after the evaporation to dryness of the decoction.

In other words, Doctor Day was able to produce a chronic form of loco poisoning with the characteristic symptoms so often described

---

[a] Presumably a 10 per cent decoction, U. S. P.

save in the occurrence of diarrhea. Diarrhea is not usually noted on the range. Sayre had already reported an ulcerated condition of the intestines of a locoed cow similar to that described by Doctor Day as occurring in cats. Doctor Day urged that the reason previous experimenters failed to produce symptoms was that they had used too small an amount of the plant and that by systematic feeding to healthy cats cases of loco disease may be produced.

Storke states that " Dr. V. C. Vaughan, of the University of Michigan, has since fully corroborated Dr. Day's views." [a]

In her experiments Doctor Day used the leaves, roots, and stems of the plants gathered in September. She believed that the greatest amount of poison is present in autumn and winter. She later undertook the isolation of the active principle, and proceeded as follows: [b]

The roots, stems, and leaves were boiled ten hours, strained, and the decoction concentrated to a sirup, poured, while hot, into a hot flask, corked and set away. At the end of ten days the sirup had separated into two layers—the upper a blackish liquid, the lower a brownish sediment. The liquid was poured into a flask and covered with six times its volume of very dilute alcohol, 30 per cent (the sediment also was washed with dilute alcohol, to insure a complete removal of the liquid), corked, and let stand three days; agitated occasionally, then filtered, and the filtrate slowly evaporated in the air, when crystals were formed. It was found important not to hurry the evaporation, for when this took place too rapidly the crystals did not form.

These crystals are microscopic in size, blue-white in color, and of a variety of forms. The most characteristic are slender and pointed, arranged in rosettes or grouped in various ways. They are soluble in distilled water and very dilute alcohol, very sparingly soluble in strong alcohol, not soluble in chloroform or ether.

The evaporated mass containing the crystals, when dissolved in distilled water, is slightly acid in reaction. A small amount of this fed to a kitten produced the train of characteristic toxic symptoms—sleepiness, loss of appetite, retching, and diarrhea—that is produced by quite large amounts of the decoction.

The crystals Sayre [c] claims to have already seen. He says that they gave no precipitate with Mayer's reagent, platinum chlorid, or with ammonia, but that barium chlorid and ammonium oxalate gave a precipitate, and he believes that they were in reality an inorganic combination of calcium, so that while Doctor Day may have obtained an extract which produced characteristic symptoms she certainly has not isolated any pure active principle. Later she admitted that it was

---

[a] Storke, B. F. The Loco Weed. Med. Current, vol. 8, p. 157. 1892.

[b] Day, M. G. The Separation of the Poison of the " Loco Weed." N. Y. Med. Journ., vol. 50, p. 604. 1889.

[c] Sayre, L. E. Active Principle of Loco Weed. Notes on New Remedies, vol. 2, No. 12, p. 1.

not possible " to make positive statements as to the chemical character of the active principle." [a]

In 1884 there was a fatal outbreak of a disorder in horses in portions of the Missouri Valley in Iowa, Nebraska, and Dakota. This
was almost uniformly fatal in a few weeks or months. The animals
lost strength and became emaciated, although they were kept in pas-
ture where there was abundant grass. There was marked stupor, the
animals falling asleep while eating, and they " would remain standing for a whole week, sleeping much of the time, with the head rest-
ing upon some object." The post-mortem examination showed that
" in every instance there was marked hemorrhagic effusion into the
fourth ventricle, the liver and spleen were abnormally dense, the walls
of the intestines were almost destitute of blood, and the stomach enormously distended with undigested food." The post-mortem find and
clinical symptoms suggested to Stalker [b] that this disorder was due to
some plant analagous to *Astragalus mollissimus*. He found abundant
in these regions *Crotalaria sagittalis*, or rattle-box, one of the so-
called loco weeds, and by the administration per os to a young horse
of an infusion of 15 pounds of the plant, given in two days, produced the clinical symptoms and the post-mortem condition of the
brain which he previously observed on the range.

.Power and Cambier [c] undertook the chemical study and the isolation of the active principle of this plant, together with that of
Astragalus mollissimus. They found that the *Astragalus mollissimus* if distilled with water yielded a distillate which possessed a
peculiar odor, which they thought due to a trace of volatile oil. On
distilling with alkali they obtained ammonia and a trace of trimethylamine. In the case of Crotalaria only ammonia was found.[d] They
argued that because trimethylamine was not obtained in this case
choline was not present. On distilling the *Astragalus mollissimus*
with acidulated water (H_2SO_4) the distillate was found to contain
acetic acid—settling the nature of the " peculiar organic acid " described by Kennedy. From this plant they obtained a resin or mixture of resinous bodies by extracting the plant with alcohol, and after
concentration precipitating with acid water. These resins in doses
of from 2 to 5 grains failed to produce any symptoms in kittens.

[a] Day, M. G. Loco Weed, in F. P. Foster's Reference-Book of Practical Therapeutics, vol. 1, p. 588. 1896.

[b] Stalker, M. 1st Ann. Rept. State Vet. Surg. Iowa, p. 16. 1885.

[c] Power, F. B., and Cambier, J. Chemical Examination of Some Loco-
Weeds. Pharm. Rundschau, vol. 9, p. 8. 1891.—Power, F. B. Notes on the
So-called Loco Weeds. Pharm. Rundschau, vol. 7, p. 134, 1889.—See also
Hoffmann, F., Loco-Weeds, in Pharm. Rundschau, vol. 7, p. 168. 1889.

[d] Kennedy, J. Pharm. Rec., vol. 8, p. 197. 1888. Kennedy also obtained ammonia from *Astragalus mollissimus*.

An albuminoid which was obtained by precipitating a concentrated aqueous extract of *Astragalus mollissimus* by means of alcohol likewise was found to be inactive to a kitten in doses corresponding to 50 grams of the crude plant. A globulin which was isolated by precipitation from a 10 per cent sodium chlorid solution proved also to be inactive in doses of 0.2 gram. They then extracted 3 kilograms of these plants with ½ per cent sulphuric acid, and after evaporation to a thick gum the mass was extracted with strong alcohol, the alcoholic solution was evaporated, and the alcoholic residue taken up in water and precipitated by neutral and basic lead acetates, and after removing the lead with sulphureted hydrogen the filtrate gave precipitates with various alkaloidal reagents. The sirupy residue which they obtained from *Astragalus mollissimus* by decomposing the precipitate with Mayer's solution administered to kittens in doses of 0.1 gram produced merely frothing at the mouth with profuse flow of saliva, but the animals soon recovered. The presence of a large amount of calcium was shown but not estimated quantitatively.

Power and Cambier summed up their conclusions by stating that both the Astragalus and the Crotalaria contain very small amounts of toxic alkaloids, to which they believe the symptoms of poisoning produced were due. Their work from a chemical standpoint is excellent, but from a pharmacological point of view seems to be deficient; in fact, Power does not claim to be a pharmacologist. What would seem to be the proper course would have been to test for themselves the action of the plant on various animals and, after deciding which reacted most characteristically, test, after various precipitations, both the precipitates and filtrates on various animals to see whether the original symptoms and pathological lesions could be produced. They failed, however, to test their mother substance. It is well recognized that plants grown under varying conditions and on different soils vary in the amount of the physiologically active principle they contain.

In the case of Crotalaria, Power and Cambier had before them the experiment of Stalker, in which he reproduced the disorder by feeding the plant extract to horses, yet they claimed that the body which they administered was the active principle, merely because it produced some frothing at the mouth and salivation in a kitten. The percentage of active principle they found would be too small to account for the symptoms, except in the case of a very active compound.

Certain of these precipitates were also later examined physiologically by O'Brine.[a] He also found the resin precipitated from an

---

[a] O'Brine, D. Progress Bulletin on the Loco and Larkspur. Colo. State Agric. Coll. Bul. 25, p. 18. 1893.

alcoholic extract of the plant and also the alcoholic extract from 2.2 pounds of the dried *Astragalus mollissimus* to be physiologically inactive.

Oatman,[a] using Power and Cambier's method with alfalfa (*Medicago sativa*), obtained a noncrystalline mass which when given in 0.1 gram dose caused frothing at the mouth in a kitten, but no serious symptoms. This 0.1 gram represented about 5 pounds of powdered leaves and tops of the plants.

Since the appearance of Power and Cambier's work Sayre has published various papers on the loco weeds in the Transactions of the Kansas Academy of Sciences for 1903–4, vol. 19, p. 194, 1905; 1901–2, vol. 18, p. 141; Seventh Biennial Report of the State Board of Agriculture of Kansas, vol. 12, p. 97, 1891; Journal of the Kansas Medical Society, vol. 4, pp. 222 and 241, 1904, etc. He has contributed nothing especially new, but says that "the old theory that an alkaloidal poison is secreted in the plant causing the loco trouble has not been found tenable," but wishes to be understood that he does not discredit the ground for the opinion that in some mysterious way certain disorders occur in cattle in connection with what is commonly called loco weed. He suggests that this connection might be somewhat similar to the relationship between the disorder caused by over-feeding half-starved animals on clover or alfalfa[b] and has had the plant analyzed as to its nutritive value, giving the table in the Transactions of the Kansas Academy of Sciences, vol. 19, p. 194. He makes the suggestion that any injurious action the plants may have might be due to the fine, hair-like projections on the plant which mechanically set up irritation. This supposition can be thrown out at once by the experiment of Day and others, who induced symptoms in animals by extracts of the plant, and by the fact that other coarse plants do not act similarly. This fine, hair-like material was found to constitute about 33 per cent of the plant on grinding. But Sayre himself does not seem to be positive as to any conclusion. He, like O'Brine and others, has obtained alkaloidal reactions from the plant, but states he has obtained similar ones from alfalfa.[c] At one time he said:

I do not consider loco directly or indirectly the cause of the condition, but am of the opinion that what is called "locoed" is, first, congestion of the brain and spinal marrow (causing blindness and first symptoms), and, second,

---

[a] Oatman, H. C. The Poisonous Principle of Loco Weed. Notes on New Remedies, vol. 4, p. 14. 1891–92.

[b] Sayre, L. E. Loco Weed. Kans. Acad. Sci. Trans., vol. 18, p. 141. 1903.

[c] Sayre, L. E. Loco Weeds. 7th Bienn. Rept. Kans. State Board Agric. for 1889–90, vol. 12, pt. 2, p. 99. 1891.

softening to a greater or less extent.[a] These terms describing the alleged symptoms of "locoism" might occur in well recognized diseases resulting from brain lesions, which latter occur in so-called forage poisoning and poisoning from foul drinking water, etc.

We are not prepared to affirm or deny that the loco weed produces a train of symptoms characteristic of the plant.[b]

Again Sayre states:

It seems not unreasonable to suppose that the peculiar condition of the animals of the plains, when they gorge themselves with this highly nitrogenous weed, has something to do with the disease. A condition of malnutrition may set in and give rise to the rapid growth of a toxic-producing micro-organism or an irritating principle. This principle may be capable of cultivation and of producing disease artificially. Be this as it may, we feel warranted in saying that the so-called poison is a development within the animal, not a product preexisting in the weed itself.

Sayre also suggests the possibility of the plants producing hydrocyanic acid, which, it is well known, occurs in sorghum.[c] In the Journal of the Kansas Medical Society (vol. 4, p. 243), he claims to have isolated a crystalline body, but this he has not tested physiologically. Sayre especially deserves credit for keeping the loco investigation alive, and no doubt his change in position is due to his lack of facilities for pharmacological testing.

Carl Ruedi[d] fed rabbits daily by a stomach tube with 10 c. c. of an extract (unstated strength) of *Astragalus mollissimus* and recorded the following results:

After only five injections one of the rabbits died, and the post-mortem showed to a nicety the congestion of the whole tract of the vena portæ and the anæmia of the brain. I put six rabbits under the influence of loco, and the effect was marked, but not rapid, if not given in very concentrated solutions. The solutions were prepared differently, and each of the rabbits had its own preparation, but the effect was nearly the same. In the beginning loco acts as a stimulant; the animals get lively, hilarious, running about, cleaning themselves, etc. This lasts about eight hours, then they become very quiet, sit in a corner of a box, and one can do with them pretty nearly what one likes; they do not move from the place, or just run into another corner, to fall back into the same complacent reverie. One can leave the door open and hammer away at the box, but they do not show any inclination to run away. During the excitement, however, they become fierce, and I had once the opportunity to watch one of the drollest things possible: One of the rabbits, two hours after dosing it, got

---

[a] Sayre, L. E. Further Report on Loco Weeds. Notes on New Remedies, vol. 4, p. 80. 1891–92.

[b] Sayre, L. E. The Loco Disease. Journ. Kans. Med. Soc., vol. 4, pp. 241–243. 1904.—What is Insanity in Lower Animals? Journ. Kans. Med. Soc., vol. 4, p. 222. 1904.

[c] Sayre, L. E. Loco Weed. Kans. Acad. Sci. Trans., vol. 18, p. 144. 1903.

[d] Ruedi, C. Loco Weed (Astragalus Mollissimus) : A Toxico-Chemical Study. Trans. Colo. State Med. Soc., p. 418. 1895.—Also Treatment of Animals Poisoned by Loco Weed (unpublished article).

loose and ran under a porch. A heavy tomcat came near this hole, and commenced sniffing about; this offended the rabbit highly, and it jumped on the neck of the cat, bit it through the skin, and the cat ran screaming away. When the animals are first under the influence of moderate doses of loco, they suffer greatly from hyperæsthesia of the cutaneous nerves; when one touches them with a stick while lying in a corner, without hurting them, one sees the platysma working away very forcibly, and sometimes they utter sounds of pain. According to my experiments the loco weed works slowly but surely; as soon as the anæmia of the brain sets in, the animals act in every respect mad like; one hour they are excitable, and then again dull and languid as can be. The rabbits eat, when well, very quickly, and whenever they have opportunity; not so the locoed rabbit; he eats slowly for a minute or two, then he goes into a corner and meditates, comes forward to nibble at a carrot or a piece of cabbage, but he never eats greedily, and does not steal it from the mouth of his neighbor, or only very exceptionally. I observed these rabbits for ten days; they did not die, because I gave them weaker solutions; but they all became very ill, and as I had to leave the park I killed them with the needle inserted into the medulla oblongata, and made the post-mortem. In all of these cases I found great congestion in the abdomen, and marked anæmia of the brain. The congestion of the vena portæ commences certainly very early, but still the first symptoms are the nervous symptoms, first as excitants, then depressing or sedative, with a marked hyperæsthesia of the cutaneous nerves.

Ruedi made an attempt to isolate the active principle and separated a base, which he calls "locoin," from an ether shaking. This base, however, he found to be physiologically inactive, but believes the activity to be due to a body which he calls " loco-acid," which is present in the mother liquid after the shaking with ether. He, however, has not obtained this in any degree of purity and gives no chemical data to substantiate this statement save that the fluid was acid.

Experiments made at the University of Pennsylvania with certain loco plants on cats, dogs, and rabbits proved negative.[a]

Other experiments on rabbits have been made by Doctor Lewis. These rabbits were fed on the leaves, stem, and whole plant, and also extracts of one of the loco plants (presumably *Astragalus mollissimus*) for one or two months, without producing any noticeable effect.[b]

This uncertainty in the results of the investigation as to the cause of the loco disease turned the attention of observers into other lines. President Ingersoll,[c] of the State Agricultural College of Colorado, in his autopsies on sheep was struck by the presence of tapeworms (*Taenia expansa*) in the gall duct and small intestines. He apparently tried to prove a relationship between the tapeworms and the locoed condition by feeding the extract of a loco plant to sheep, and thus showing its harmlessness. He prepared a decoction from 20 pounds of loco plant

---

[a] The " Loco Disease."   Therap. Gaz., vol. 12, p. 30.   1888.

[b] Sayre, L. E.   Loco Weed.   Kans. Acad. Sci. Trans., vol. 18, p. 142.   1903.

[c] Sayre, L. E.   Loco Weeds.   7th Bien. Rept. Kansas State Board Agric. for 1889–1890, pt. 2, p. 98.   1891.

(the species was not stated) and boiled this down from 12 gallons to 1 quart. This concentrated extract was fed in three days to a bottle-fed lamb; this lamb showed no symptoms, although kept under observation for two weeks. This theory of the causation of loco by worms was also considered by Curtice,[a] and later brought forward by Steele [b] and Marshall.[c] This idea is very suggestive when considered in relation to the etiology of bothriocephalous anæmia.[d]

Others, again, have claimed that the disease is due to a parasite found upon the loco plants, but all specimens examined by entomologists proved to be harmless.[e]

Lloyd, from his study of the subject, says:

From first to last I have failed in obtaining a characteristic proximate principle, either from the fresh or dried plant. The disease called loco was as murky as the milk sickness so prevalent in the new settlements of Indiana and Kentucky in early days, and, like the numberless herbs that have been presumed to produce that obscure peculiar disease, milk sickness, loco was unresponsive to my chemistry.[f]

It may be safely said that if a specimen of the plant were to be examined in the ordinary manner by a chemist who had no idea of its importance he would report that it did not contain a characteristic proximate constituent.[g]

Can it be that an admixture of loco and some undetermined plant or earth infected with bacteria taken with the roots, each innocuous under other conditions, can by digestion together in the stomach and intestines result in the production of a poison?[h]

To sum up, it seems to the writer that the poison of loco is a product, and not an educt.[i]

[a] Curtice, C. Tape-Worm Disease of Sheep of the Western Plains. Bur. Animal Industry, 4th and 5th Ann. Rept., p. 167. 1889.

[b] Steele, C. D. New Theory about Loco. Farm and Ranch, vol. 20, No. 35, p. 1. 1901.

[c] Marshall, H. T. Loco Weed Disease of Sheep. Johns Hopkins Hospital Bul., vol. 15, p. 181. 1904.—Data as to these parasites of sheep may be found in Curtice, C., The Animal Parasites of Sheep. Bur. Animal Industry, Rept., 1890.

[d] Faust, E. S., and Tallquist, T. W. Ueber d. Ursachen der Bothriocephalusanämie. Arch. f. Exp. Path., vol. 57, p. 367. 1907.

[e] Walshia Amorphella and the Loco Weed. Insect Life, vol. 2, p. 50. 1889–90. Snow, F. H. Loco-Weed. Science, vol. 9, p. 92. 1887.

[f] Lloyd, J. U. Loco, or Crazy Weed. Eclectic Med. Journ., vol. 53, p. 482. 1893.

[g] Lloyd, J. U., l. c., p. 483.

[h] Lloyd, J. U., l. c., p. 484.

Note.—Eccles had previously announced a somewhat similar idea. Sayre, L. E. Loco Weed. Proc. Amer. Pharm. Assoc., vol. 36, p. 115. 1889.

[i] Lloyd, J. U., l. c., p. 486.

But Lloyd adds, in speaking of the reports of various experts and ranchmen:

Their description concerning its toxic action on animals agreed, and it was folly to argue that so many observers from so many sections of the country could be misled. There must be an undetermined something behind the loco weed.[a]

In 1893 O'Brine, from Colorado, and Mayo, from Kansas, reported on their work with the loco plants. O'Brine failed to isolate any alkaloidal or other poisonous body, and his feeding experiments on himself and on rabbits having failed, he sums up in despair: " The more I examine the loco question, the more I am persuaded that we must look for some other cause besides the loco weed." [b] At the end of his report he gives some ash analyses but fails to interpret them. He also fails to give details as to the method of obtaining and estimating his ash. O'Brine's ash analyses are as follows:

Plant.	Total ash.	SiO_2.	Fe_2O_3 and Al_2O_3.	CaO.	MgO.	K_2O.	Na_2O.	H_2SO_4.	Cl.	P_2O_5.	CO_2.
Astragalus mollissimus (whole plant)	12.15	32.77	16.26	6.05	3.11	13.30	3.21	3.9	0.47	6.12	10.55
Aragallus lamberti (whole plant)	13.52	17.08	12.21	14.27	2.62	17.26	5.75	3.22	3.87	3.30	17.87
Astragalus caryocarpus	12.36	7.82	5.97	12.10	3.55	23.35	3.38	5.56	9.0	4.67	20.62

These analyses are evidently incorrect, as O'Brine estimates a carbon content of 4.13 per cent for the first, and for the second 2.22 per cent, showing incomplete combustion.

Mayo [c] experimented with alcoholic and aqueous extracts of dried *Astragalus mollissimus* on guinea pigs, with negative results, and was first led to deny a relationship between the disease and the plants. Later, as a result of the post-mortem findings, he was convinced that his first conclusion was wrong and that " the disease is certainly the result of animals feeding upon the loco weed." Mayo says:

A careful survey of the experiments performed and observations noted leads me to the opinion that the disease known as " loco " is the result of malnutrition, or a gradual starvation, caused by the animals eating the plants known as " loco weeds," either *Astragalus mollissimus* or *Aragallus lamberti.* If there is a narcotic principle in the plant, chemists have failed to find it and a fluid extract does not possess it, and a ton of the plant eaten by an animal ought to contain enough of the poisonous properties to destroy an animal.

[a] Lloyd, J. U., l. c., p. 483.

[b] O'Brine, D. Progress Bulletin on the Loco and Larkspur. Colo. State Agric. Coll. Bul. 25, p. 17. 1893.

[c] Mayo, N. S. Some Observations on Loco. Kans. State Agric. Coll. Bul. 35, p. 116. 1893.

Kobert.[a] has also tested the activity of *Astragalus mollissimus* and says. " Ich fand *Astragalus mollissimus* ziemlich unwirksam."

Doctor McEackran [b] fed dried *Astragalus mollissimus* and *Aragallus lamberti* mixed with feed to a stabled animal for two months without result. (Animal not stated).[c] Similar negative experiments are reported from the State of Washington. but the amounts used were too small to form any conclusions.[d]

Mr. V. K. Chesnut [e] has busied himself with the loco problem. but mainly in an executive capacity, his own efforts being directed to the study of the relation of the loco plants to the disease on the range. He has done no laboratory work. Chesnut and Wilcox made numerous autopsies on sheep and experiments on animals. They claimed that an extract of *Aragallus spicatus* produced some slight narcotic action in rabbits. Their pathological examinations failed to show any characteristic lesion. but they state that the cerebral membranes were in all cases slightly congested. They deny any causative relationship to the presence of worms or with feeding upon alkalis. They believe that sheep are more likely to become locoed if not salted regularly. Chesnut describes one case in which a lamb became locoed by nursing from a locoed mother.

In 1901 Reid Hunt. at that time a special agent of the United States Department of Agriculture. studied the loco question in Montana. working mainly with *Aragallus spicatus*. He moistened the ground-up plant with 93 per cent ethyl alcohol and then percolated it until exhausted. This extract was evaporated and taken up with water so that 1 c. c. of the solution corresponded to 10 grams of the plant. This was fed to an active young rabbit weighing 490 grams, 6 c. c. being fed by the mouth and followed in about an hour by 10 c. c. more, and two hours after this by 15 c. c. This rabbit showed no symptoms during the following day. The next day it was very dull and there was marked muscular weakness, as the rabbit's legs were spread wide apart and his nose rested on the ground. Later respiration became very slow and the pupils were dilated. The paralytic symptoms increased and finally. after a convulsive movement. the

---

[a] Kobert, R. Lehrb. d. Intoxikationen, p. 615. 1893.

[b] O'Brine, D. Progress Bulletin on Loco and Larkspur. Colo. State Agric. Coll. Bul. 25, p. 13. 1893.

[c] After the manuscript of this bulletin was sent to the printer it was learned through Professor Carpenter that this animal was a horse.

[d] Nelson, S. B. Feeding Wild Plants to Sheep. Bur. Animal Industry, Bul. 22, p. 12. 1898.

[e] Chesnut. V. K., and Wilcox. E. V. Stock-Poisoning Plants of Montana. U. S. Dept. Agric., Div. Bot., Bul. 26, p. 95. 1901.—Wilcox, E. V. Plant Poisoning of Stock in Montana. Bur. Animal Industry. 17th Ann. Rept.. p. 111. 1900.

NOTE.—The writer wishes to acknowledge the great literary help Mr. Chesnut's card catalogue has been to him in the preparation of this paper.

animal died, thirty-six hours after the first feeding. Hunt merely states of the post-mortem examination that the stomach was well filled and that the " walls seem normal."

Hunt tried to isolate an active principle by the Dragendorff method, but failed to obtain any physiologically active shakings. He tried hypodermic injections of 80 per cent alcohol extractions of the fresh green plant, and after the injection of an extract corresponding to 60 grams of the fresh plant there was no effect produced. He tried to induce symptoms by feeding the plant itself to rabbits, but was unsuccessful, as the rabbits refused to eat the plant. He was not able to induce symptoms with the extracts of the dried plant.[a]

Marshall [b] studied the loco question with regard to sheep and practically denies the existence of a locoed condition due to eating the loco plants, but believes the condition due to bad feeding, parasitism, etc. He lays great stress upon the presence of worms, but fails to see that they may be merely a secondary infection superimposed upon an already morbid condition produced by eating the plants. Others have claimed that the cause is an insect living upon the loco plants. Others, again, have suggested an analogy with trypanosome disorders.

Chesnut has held the view that many of the cases of so-called locoed sheep were really due to parasites, but that there was a true locoed condition due to eating the loco weeds.

The lack of agreement in the results of the investigators has caused many to doubt any positive relation between the plant and the disease, and even as late as 1904 Payne [c] practically says these diseases are due to lack of nutrition and not to the loco plant. The matter has been summed up in a recent work as follows:

> Though many chemists have sought for the constituents, none have been able to locate the active properties, the trace of alkaloids, resins, volatile and fixed oils having each in turn been found destitute of it. Yet the poisonous properties are fully established by field observations. The destructiveness of these plants to stock is so great as to have probably caused upward of a million dollars loss in the aggregate, and large bounties have been offered by State governments for an effective method of avoiding such losses. It is considered very probable that the poisonous constituent is albuminoidal.[d]

---

[a] Unpublished report.

[b] Marshall, H. T. Loco Weed Disease of Sheep. Johns Hopkins Hospital Bul., vol. 15, p. 182. 1904.

[c] Payne, J. E. Cattle Raising on the Plains. Colo. Agric. Expt. Sta. Bul. 87, p. 16. 1904.

[d] National Standard Dispensatory, p. 868. 1905.

NOTE.—The field experiments of Harding and Tudor are rather conclusive as to the relation of these plants to this disorder. Sayre, L. E., Loco Weed, Amer. Vet. Rev., vol. 11, pp. 553–554, 1887—Blankinship, J. W., Loco and Some Other Poisonous Plants in Montana, Mont. Agric. Exper. Sta. Bul. 45, pp. 83–84, 1903—Loco Disease, Therap. Gaz., vol. 12, p. 30, 1898.

NOTES ON VARIOUS MEMBERS OF THE LOCO-WEED FAMILY.

Astragalus caryocarpus is at times eaten in some of the Western States. but is claimed by some at certain stages of its growth to contain a poisonous principle. Frankforter,[a] from experiments on himself. however, denies this.

Astragalus glycophyllus has been used as a diuretic and *Astragalus exscapus* in the treatment of syphilis.[b] "The seed of *A. boeticus*, planted in Germany and England, are found to be the very best substitute for coffee yet tried, and so used—roasted, parched, and mixed with coffee."[c] *Astragalus nuttallianus*, according to Smith,[d] is a highly nutritious forage plant in spring. *Astragalus crassicarpus* has been prophesied by him to be a valuable addition to early spring soiling crops. *Astragalus adsurgens* (*nitidus*) and one or two other species of Astragalus are still used in Chinese medicine.[e] The Indians of the Southwest are familiar with certain loco plants.[f] The Tewans of Hano are said to eat the root of *Aragallus lamberti*, and *Astragalus mollissimus* is applied locally for headaches by some of the Arizona Indians. One of these species is used as a flavoring material by the Coahuillas and is mixed with other plants as spices.[g] *Astragalus kentrophyta* had a reputation among the Navajos for the treatment of rabies.[h] The use of certain loco plants—*Astragalus mollissimus*—has been advocated on theoretical grounds in the treatment of certain forms of insanity, but without favorable results.[i] In Peru and Chile *Astragalus garbancillo*, *A. unifultus*, and *A. ochroleucus* have been considered injurious to animals.[j] *Astragalus glyciphyllus* and *A. alpinus* have been used in Europe as food for stock.[k]

---

[a] Frankforter, G. B. A Chemical Study of Astragalus Caryocarpus. Amer. Journ. Pharm., vol. 72, p. 320. 1900.

[b] Maisch. J. M. Poisonous Species of Astragalus. Amer. Journ. Pharm., vol. 51, p. 240. 1879.—Fleurot. Chimiques et Pharmaceutiques sur la Racines d'Astragale sans Tiges. Journ. de Chim. Med., vol. 10. p. 656. 1834.

[c] Porcher, F. P. Resources of the Southern Fields and Forests, p. 204. 1869.

[d] Smith, J. G. Fodder and Forage Plants. U. S. Dept. Agric., Div. Agrost., Bul. 2 (rev. ed.), p. 12. 1900.

[e] Holmes. E. M. Notes on Chinese Drugs. Pharm. Journ. and Trans., vol. 21, 3 s., p. 1149. 1891.

[f] Hough, W. Environmental Interrelations in Arizona. Amer. Anthropologist, vol. 11, pp. 143, 147. 1898.

[g] Barrows. D. P. Ethno-Botany of the Coahuilla Indians of Southern California, p. 67. 1900.

[h] Matthews, W. Navajo Names for Plants. Amer. Nat., vol. 20, p. 772. 1886.

[i] Givens, A. J. Loco or Crazy Weed. Med. Century. vol. 1. p. 21. 1893.—Compare Hurd, H. M. Amer. Journ. Insanity. vol. 42, p. 178. 1885-86.

. [j] Rosenthal. D. A. Synopsis Plantarum Diaphoricarum, Erlangen. 1861, p. 1004. Greshoff, M. Beschrijving d. Giftige en Bedwelmende Planten bij de Vischvangst in Gebruik, p. 51. 1900.

[k] Pott, E. Handb. d. tierisch. Ernährung, vol. 2, p. 113. 1907.

Details as to the use of other Astragali can be found in Planchon, G., Sur les Astragales, in Journal de Pharmacie et de Chimie, 5th series, vol 24, p. 473, 1891; 5th series, vol. 25, pp. 169, 233, 1892.

LABORATORY EXPERIMENTS—PHYSIOLOGICAL.

The first point in our investigations was to determine whether the plant exerted any poisonous action and to find some animal which responded regularly to it; then to ascertain if the lack of results of previous investigators was not due to insufficient doses, and later to see if by feeding smaller amounts at repeated intervals symptoms comparable to those described as occurring on the range could not be produced. The animal finally selected was the rabbit.

EXPERIMENTS ON RABBITS.

ACUTE CASES.

Experiment No. 1.—On September 8, 1905, an aqueous extract of 333 grams of fresh *Astragalus mollissimus*, made in Hugo, Colo., and shipped preserved in chloroform,[a] killed a rabbit weighing 1,616 grams in one hour and thirty-five minutes, while an extract corresponding to 167 grams merely caused drowsiness and loss of appetite in a rabbit weighing 765 grams.

Experiment No. 2.—On November 29, 1905, a rabbit weighing 1,162.3 grams was fed with a concentrated aqueous extract of 500 grams of fresh *Astragalus mollissimus*, which had been shipped from Hugo, Colo., preserved in chloroform in sealed vessels. This animal died in one hour and ten minutes. The symptoms consisted in dullness, rapid respiration, and signs of pain. At autopsy the stomach and upper part of the small intestines showed hemorrhagic ecchymoses, with dilation of the dural vessels of the brain and cord, with a clot over a portion of the spinal cord.

Experiment No. 3.—On February 13, 1906, a rabbit weighing 992 grams was fed with a concentrated aqueous extract of 500 grams of the fresh *Astragalus mollissimus*, collected in September and preserved in chloroform water. Before feeding, the rabbit's ears were warm and the rabbit struggled when any attempt was made to turn him on his back. The temperature at 10.50 a. m., the time of feeding, was 103.5° F.; at 11.15 a. m., 102.5° F. At 11.30 a. m. the rabbit was breathing very rapidly and would stay on his back for some time if

---

[a] In all cases in which the plants were preserved with chloroform sealed vessels were used for shipping. The chloroform was carefully evaporated off in vacuo before feeding the extract, the evaporation requiring several hours. The plants were collected by Dr. C. Dwight Marsh, in charge of the field investigations at Hugo, Colo.

placed so. The temperature at this time was 102.6° F. Both pupils, the one exposed to the light and the one protected, were contracted. At 12.02 p. m. convulsive movements of the legs appeared. The rabbit made one leap, the temperature rose to 103.6° F., and after a few convulsive movements of the limbs the anus relaxed and a small stool appeared, the pupils dilated, and the animal died at 12.06 p. m.

Experiment No. 4.—The feeding of the extract of 464 grams induced a fall in temperature of 2.4° F. in three hours, and the rabbit died several hours later (at night).

Experiment No. 5.—March 2, 1906, a rabbit weighing 928 grams was fed with a concentrated extract of 500 grams of the fresh seeds and pods of *Astragalus mollissimus*, made in September, 1905, and preserved with chloroform water. This animal died in one hour and seven minutes. The animal showed the usual post-mortem conditions.

It was thus found that the aqueous extract of 500 grams of the fresh *Astragalus mollissimus* would cause death in about one hour in rabbits weighing about 2 pounds (907 grams), these rabbits showing constant clinical symptoms—urination, paralysis, more or less convulsive muscular twitchings, often terminating in general convulsions, drowsiness, and stupor, with more or less anesthesia. The pupils at the time of death were often unequal. At first there was usually a slight rise in temperature, but this was soon succeeded by a fall. Often there were soft stools. The post-mortem lesions in these cases were marked congestion, with hemorrhages in the stomach walls and a secretion of thick mucus. The portions of the stomach walls most affected were the dependent portions near the cardiac end. The intestines showed dilatation of the blood vessels. The mesenteric vessels and also the vessels in the cerebral portions of the dura were markedly dilated; in some cases there were clots, especially at the posterior portion of the brain, between the cerebrum and the cerebellum. At times there were clots over the dorsal portion of the cord. On cutting into the brain the brain substance itself did not appear to be congested. The cord seemed about normal, but the vessels of its membranes were well marked. The other organs showed nothing characteristic macroscopically. These experiments were repeated many times and found to be constant.

These acute symptoms were likewise produced by an extract of 500 grams of the fresh *Aragallus lamberti* from Arizona preserved in chloroform water (rabbit weighing 1,998 grams). An aqueous extract of 150 grams of the dried *Astragalus mollissimus*[a] from Imperial, Nebr. (1906), caused death in one hour and fifty-eight minutes

---

[a] All extracts from dried material were made at Washington.

in a rabbit weighing 1,530 grams, and an extract of 100 grams killed in one hour and twenty-two minutes a rabbit weighing 736 grams.

An aqueous extract of 100 grams of the dried *Astragalus bigelowii* induced death in one hour and thirty-eight minutes, the rabbit weighing 1,502 grams.

An aqueous extract of 150 grams of *Astragalus nitidus* collected at Woodland Park, Colo., in 1906 induced death in three hours and five minutes, the rabbit weighing 1,672 grams.

An aqueous extract of 200 grams of the dried *Astragalus bisulcatus* caused death after several hours (at night), the rabbit weighing 2,423 grams.

In certain cases this production of acute symptoms was not entirely a question of salt action, as was shown by certain other experiments. In other cases salt action seems to be the important factor, so that the production of these acute symptoms can not always be considered characteristic.

CHRONIC CASES.

Experiment No. 6.—February 19, 1906, a large gray rabbit weighing 2,055.3 grams was fed with 60 c. c. of fluid representing the concentrated aqueous extract of 250 grams of the fresh *Astragalus mollissimus*, collected September 18, 1905, and preserved in chloroform. This rabbit was very hard to hold. The ears rested on the body. The temperature at the time of feeding, 1.30 p. m., was 102.3° F. At 2.57 p. m. the animal looked dull but resisted handling. At 3.30 p. m. it urinated. At 4.15 p. m. the temperature was 98.5° F., the pupils were about the same size as before feeding, and the animal became much duller. The next day at 12.50 p. m. the temperature was 102.4° F., and at this time the animal could be handled with greater ease. The animal ate in the morning. The same amount of extract was again fed at 1.24 p. m. At 1.35 p. m. the animal was much duller and could be turned on his back with ease. If disturbed he ran against the wall as if utterly unconscious of the obstruction. The animal had soft, liquid, brown stools and tried to lie down as much as possible. If turned on its back with the feet up it would stay so almost indefinitely. Temperature, 103.8° F.; respiration very rapid. At 2.40 p. m. the temperature was 99.8° F., and the animal died a few minutes later. After death the pupils were much contracted. The vessels of the dura covering the brain were much dilated, but the vessels inside the brain were not dilated. The stomach walls were congested and marked with numerous petechiæ and covered with mucus.

Experiment No. 7.—On February 19, 1906, a white and brown rabbit whose temperature was 103.2° F. was fed 30 c. c. of aqueous fluid representing the concentrated extract of 125 grams of the fresh

Astragalus mollissimus, collected September, 1905, and preserved with chloroform. The rabbit weighed 1,502.5 grams. This extract was fed at 1.45 p. m., and at 4.15 p. m. the temperature was 102.6° F., but there were no marked symptoms. The following day at 2.04 p. m. the temperature registered 102.5° F. The same amount of extract was given at 2.09 p. m. The temperature at 4 p. m. was 99.8° F., the animal was dull, and the pupils were perhaps a little smaller. The animal could not be turned over without resistance. The following day, February 21, at 1.30 p. m. the temperature was 102.6° F., and at 1.45 the same amount of extract was given. At 1.54 p. m. the animal was much duller and the breathing was very rapid. At 4.10 p. m. the temperature was 101.3° F. The animal had been dull ever since the feeding was begun. It nibbled food shortly before the last feeding. On February 23 the same amount of extract was given at 2.16 p. m., temperature 99° F. The breathing was very rapid, the ears shaking, and there was a sleepy, dull look about the animal. At 3.30 p. m. the animal was dull, but would still walk about if disturbed. At this time the animal weighed 1,445.8 grams. At 4.30 p. m. the temperature was 102° F. and the pupils were about normal size. There was a marked sleepy look about the animal, which sat quietly in its cage.

February 24, at 1 p. m., the animal was very dull and could with ease be turned on its back with its feet in the air. It would sit in its cage perfectly quiet. The weight at this time was 1,417.5 grams, the temperature 96.6° F. On February 26 the animal weighed 1,360.8 grams. It was dull and refused to eat. The abdomen felt very distended and tympanitic. February 27 the weight was still 1,360.8 grams, and the animal sat in its cage as if asleep, with eyes half closed. There was no diarrhea and the abdomen was very distended. At 11.15 a. m. there was a general convulsion and the animal fell over. At 12 m. the abdomen seemed even more swollen, the animal was hardly able to walk, and it fell over, uttering a cry. Pupils were about normal—perhaps a little smaller. The animal died at 12.10 p. m.

The post-mortem, made immediately after death, showed the abdomen markedly tympanitic, and the large intestines could be outlined through the abdominal walls with ease. The large intestines were of a chocolate color, intensely congested, and marked with hemorrhages. On opening the abdomen there was a decided putrefactive odor, and about an ounce of bloody fluid was found in the peritoneal cavity, together with fibrin flakes. The stomach was pale, the first three inches of the small intestine up to where it turned sharply were pale, and below this the intestines were injected and full of gas and of a dark red color. The kidneys were 3½ centimeters long and were pale, capsules easily peeled off; cortex pale. Liver pale and infected with some coccideæ. The gall bladder was one-quarter inch wide and one inch long. Spleen a trifle pale; lungs pale, nothing abnormal; heart relaxed. On opening the stomach gas and fluid, with some food, exuded. The walls were pale, but pink in some places. There was no marked congestion or hemorrhage or perforation. The mesenteric vessels were dilated. The upper portion of the intestines contained a little mucus-like fluid, but lower down became bloody, and still lower contained pus-like fluid. The walls were hemorrhagic. The large intestine contained a soft, fecal-like fluid, very foul. Its walls were much congested and full of hemorrhagic points. The cortex of the suprarenal bodies was sharply defined, the medullæ brownish. Brain pale, some dural vessels well marked, no clots or hemorrhages. Base of brain pale. No congestion seen on cutting into the brain. Spinal cord showed no hemorrhages or lymph effusions.

Experiment No. 8.—On February 18, 1906, at 2 p. m., a rabbit whose temperature was 102.2° F. was fed with the aqueous extract of 125 grams of fresh *Astragalus mollissimus*, collected in September, 1905, and preserved in chloroform, 30 c. c. of the fluid being used. At 4.25 p. m. the temperature was 102.4° F. No symptoms were noted. This rabbit weighed 1,644.3 grams. On February 20 at 2.09 p. m. the temperature was 102.2° F. and the rabbit showed no symptoms. The same dose was repeated at 2.15 p. m. At 4 p. m. the temperature was 100.3° F. The rabbit was dull but could not be turned over without a struggle. February 21 at 1.30 p. m. the temperature was 101.4° F. The same amount of extract was fed at 1.45 p. m. At this time the animal was dull and breathed more rapidly. At 4.10 p. m. the temperature was 97.3° F. Next day the same amount of extract was again given at 2 p. m. At 2.16 p. m. the breathing became rapid and the animal duller. The ears were directed forward. At 4.15 p. m. the temperature was 101.6° F.; weight 1,757.7 grams; animal slightly dull. February 24, temperature 102° F., weight 1,786 grams. March 5, weight 1,729.3 grams. The animal was fed at 3.20 p. m. with a concentrated extract of 125 grams of *Astragalus mollissimus*, collected in September. Temperature at time of feeding 100.4° F.; 3.40 p. m., no symptoms; 4 p. m., temperature 102° F. March 7, weight 1,644.3 grams; March 8, weight 1,672.6 grams; March 10, weight 1,701 grams; March 12, weight 1,658.4 grams; March 14, weight 1,701 grams.

In this case, where the same dose was given in a period of five days, very little effect on the rabbit was noted.

Experiment No. 9.—On March 1, 1906, a black rabbit weighing 2,664.8 grams was fed with a concentrated aqueous extract of 250 grams of fresh *Astragalus mollissimus*, collected in the fall of 1905.

On March 5 the weight was 2,296.3 grams. The animal was then given the same amount of extract. During the afternoon it passed mucus and thick pieces of feces and was dull; respiration very rapid. March 6, weight 2,282 grams; March 7, 3 p. m., animal very dull and would not eat: sat hunched up, but resisted being disturbed; weight 2,310.5 grams. March 8, weight 2,183 grams; March 9, weight 2,069.5 grams. Pupils dilated; finger could be run almost against the eye, provided the lashes were not touched, without the animal winking or paying any attention. Rabbit ate very little and had not urinated since the preceding day. Left ear had fallen to the side as if the animal were unable to support it. Weight, 1,912.8 grams. From March 9 to March 11, 67 c. c. of cloudy urine were voided. This did not clear with acetic acid. Left eye tearing. March 10, head held to right side. March 12, weight 1,786 grams. Left pupil smaller than right, neither responding to light. Rabbit very weak. March 14, weight 1,729.3 grams. Would not eat. March 16, weight 1,644.3 grams. Right pupil larger than left, neither responding to light. Diarrhea present. Breathing noisy. In sitting down she raised herself on her forelegs, evidently to take the pressure off her abdomen, which was distended. If disturbed, she would butt against the side of the cage, apparently oblivious of its presence. Knee jerks were very active, almost a clonus. Reflex from tendo Achillis active. March 17, forelegs spread out, head falling to left side. The temperature had fallen below 94° F. and would not register on the ordinary clinical thermometer. The ears twitched, the head was thrown back, the abdomen was distended, and the rabbit gritted its teeth. Died. Weight, 1,559.2 grams.

Brain and spinal cord pale. Dural vessels plainly seen but not marked. Intestinal vessels congested. Stomach pale; nothing apparent macroscopically save a small pin-point ulcer.[a] Heart relaxed. Post-mortem examination otherwise negative macroscopically.

Experiment No. 10.—A mouse-colored rabbit weighing 1,927.8 grams was fed February 18, 1906, at 2.26 p. m., with a concentrated aqueous extract of 250 grams of fresh *Astragalus mollissimus* collected in September, 1905, and preserved in chloroform water. The temperature of this rabbit was 102.6° F. The fluid given was 40 c. c. At 2.45 p. m. the rabbit urinated and at 2.57 p. m. was dull and the respiration became rapid. The animal then aborted and had three young, two of which showed some movement after birth, but were apparently premature.

---

[a] Compare Plönius, W., Beziehungen d. Geschwürs u. d. Erosionen d. Magens z. d. funktionell. Störungen u. Krankh. d: Darmes, Arch. f. Verdauungsk., vol. 13, pp. 180, 270, 1907, and Tixier, L., Anémies Exper. Conséc. aux Ulcér. du Pylore, Comp. Rend. Hebd. Soc. de Biol., vol. 62, p. 1041, 1907.

On February 23 the temperature of this rabbit was 102.9° F. at 1.40 p. m. She was then fed with the same amount of the extract as before. At 2.16 p. m. she lay down and became much duller; left ear fallen to side. At 3.30 p. m. the rabbit was unable to stand. The pupil of the eye exposed to the light was dilated. The animal died without a struggle. The stomach contained much bloody mucus. In the dependent portion of the stomach near the cardiac end were marked petechiæ in the walls, with bright-red blood in the stomach itself. The heart was relaxed. The intestines showed nothing abnormal. The dural vessels of the brain were dilated; there was a clot on the dura over the fourth ventricle. Spinal cord and kidneys normal, the capsules not adhering. Weight, 1,786 grams at death.

Experiment No. 11.—On March 1, 1906, a rabbit weighing 2,126.2 grams was fed with a concentrated aqueous extract of 250 grams of the fresh *Aragallus lamberti* preserved in chloroform water. On March 5 this dose was repeated, 37.5 c. c. of the fluid being used. March 6 the rabbit weighed 1,956 grams; March 7, 1,913.6 grams; March 8, 1,828.5 grams; March 9, 1,701 grams; March 12, 1,672.6 grams; March 14, 1,644.3 grams.

Experiment No. 12.—January 19, 1906, a concentrated aqueous extract of 500 grams of the fresh *Aragallus lamberti* preserved with chloroform water was fed to a rabbit weighing 785 grams. The temperature at 12.10 p. m., the time of feeding, was 101.6° F. The temperature 1 hour and 43 minutes later was 94.6° F., and the animal died shortly after, showing the same condition as occurred after feeding extracts of *Astragalus mollissimus.*

PREGNANT ANIMALS.

Experiment No. 13.—A large, gray, pregnant rabbit weighing 2,891.6 grams was fed on February 22, 1906, with 42 c. c. of fluid, corresponding to the aqueous extract of 250 grams of *Astragalus mollissimus* collected in September and October, 1905, and preserved with chloroform. At 4 p. m. the animal was dull, but still resisted efforts to handle. On February 24 this animal weighed 2,778.2 grams, and on February 26 it bore a litter of seven young rabbits. One or two of these showed movements of the limbs, but were apparently immature. This rabbit on March 10 weighed 2,537.3 grams; March 12, 2,438 grams; March 14, 2,508.9 grams; March 22, 2,494.7 grams.

Experiment No. 14.—On March 1, 1906, a black rabbit weighing 2,721.6 grams was fed at 12.15 p. m. with a concentrated aqueous extract of 250 grams of the fresh *Astragalus mollissimus* collected in September, 1905. On March 2 it weighed 2,438 grams; at 2.58 p. m. it still resisted efforts to turn it on its back; at 3.15 p. m. it could be turned on its back with ease. March 6 the weight was 2,338.8 grams;

March 7 the animal was very dull, would not eat, pupils dilated, hind legs paralyzed; died during the night; weight, 2,267.9 grams.

The stomach walls were pale save at the dependent portion near the cardiac end, where there was a hemorrhagic, ulcerated area about 1½ by 1½ inches. The intestines were full of gas, but not hemorrhagic. The uterus contained eight immature fœti. The uterine walls were hemorrhagic. The kidneys weighed 9½ grams; their medullæ were dark and the straight tubules well defined. The cerebral dural vessels were congested and the spinal dural vessels were well defined. The bladder was found contracted. The blood gave no bands for methæmoglobin, but showed merely those of oxyhæmoglobin on spectroscopic examination.

Experiment No. 15.—Control experiments made by feeding water were negative, except when a large quantity (150 c. c.) of water was given to a rabbit weighing 1,020.5 grams. The animal died in 12 hours with marked pallor of the tissues (hydræmia), a pathological condition quite different from that obtained by feeding extracts of the loco plants, and no such results were secured with the amount of water used in our feeding experiments. 50 to 70 c. c.

SUBCUTANEOUS INJECTIONS.

Experiment No. 16.—On February 28, 1906, a white rabbit weighing 581.2 grams was injected subcutaneously at 10.35 a. m. with a concentrated aqueous extract of 83 grams of fresh *Astragalus mollissimus* collected in September, 1905, and preserved with chloroform. The temperature before injection was 102.1° F. At 1.40 p. m. the animal was dull; at 3.12 p. m. the temperature registered 99.8° F. The animal died during the night. The post-mortem examination was negative. Stomach pale; heart relaxed save left ventricle, which seemed contracted; dural vessels of the brain dilated; kidneys perhaps normal. No microscopical examination.

Experiment No. 17.—February 28, 1906, at 10.25 a. m., a guinea pig weighing 496 grams was injected subcutaneously with a concentrated aqueous extract of 83 grams of the fresh *Astragalus mollissimus* preserved in chloroform water. At 1.40 p. m. there was muscular twitching. The animal was dull and could be easily turned on his back. The hind legs began to show weakness. At 1.50 p. m. the hind legs were almost completely paralyzed and the animal could be easily turned on his back. Muscles of the limbs twitched and semen was expelled. Animal died at 2.15 p. m.

Post-mortem showed dural vessels of cord and brain full of blood. Stomach pinker than normal; mesenteric vessels dilated. Heart almost empty of blood. Kidneys congested.

129

These experiments indicate that an acute form of poisoning may be induced by feeding concentrated aqueous extracts of *Astragalus mollissimus* and *Aragallus lamberti* from Hugo, Colo., and Imperial, Nebr., to rabbits, and that if the extract is given in smaller and repeated doses a more prolonged or chronic condition may follow.

The rabbits showing the chronic effects of these plants exhibit symptoms which have a marked parallelism with those reported as occurring in larger herbivora (horses and cattle) on the range when locoed; that is, the loss of appetite (Experiment No. 9), the emaciation and loss in weight (Experiment No. 9), the dullness and stupor, with more or less anesthesia (Experiment No. 7), the disturbance in the visual function (Experiment No. 9), and the mental symptoms (Experiment No. 6). The occasional abortion compares with what has been observed in larger animals. The dried *Astragalus mollissimus* and *Aragallus lamberti* still retained their poisonous properties, as we were able to kill with aqueous extracts of the dried plants made in the laboratory under the proper conditions.

EXPERIMENTS ON SHEEP.

Experiment No. 1.—On May 31, 1906, a sheep weighing 32.2 kilos was fed with a concentrated aqueous extract of 1,000 grams of the fresh *Astragalus mollissimus* preserved in chloroform water. The temperature at 11 o'clock, the time of feeding, was 103.4° F. At 11.45 a. m. this dose was repeated. At 12 o'clock the temperature was 104.1° F. At 12.45 the animal urinated. At 1.10 p. m. a similar extract of 2,000 grams was fed. The total liquid used was 1,500 c. c. On June 1 no symptoms were noted. On June 5 an extract of 3,000 grams of fresh *Aragallus lamberti* and 3,000 grams of *Astragalus mollissimus* was fed. After feeding this the animal could be easily turned over on its back and its ear pricked with impunity. The animal at this time weighed 30.8 kilos. On June 6, at 11 a. m., the temperature was 104° F. The sheep had numerous soft stools, and was very dull, and would not eat. On June 7 the temperature was 103.7° F. and the sheep still refused to eat. On the 8th the temperature was 103.2° F. at 10.40 a .m., and the stools were still numerous and soft.

There were then fed 640 c. c., representing the aqueous extract of 4,000 grams of the fresh *Aragallus lamberti*. The animal could be easily turned on its back. It weighed at this time 28.57 kilos. On June 9, at 10.47 a. m., the temperature was 103.4° F. The sheep still did not eat, but had no diarrhea. It now weighed 27.9 kilos, and the temperature was 103° F. at 10.45 a. m.

129

On June 13 the animal began to eat, and 1,700 c. c. of fluid, representing 5,500 grams of the fresh *Aragallus lamberti*, were fed. The temperature at 12.30 p. m. was 103° F. On June 14 the temperature was 103.4° F., the animal weighed 28.3 kilos, and refused food. On June 16 the weight was 28.3 kilos; the temperature at 2 p. m. was 103.5° F. There was no diarrhea.

On June 19 the aqueous extract of 1,000 grams of the dried *Astragalus mollissimus* was fed with 420 c. c. of water. The temperature was 102.6° F. On June 20 the temperature was 102.9° F. at 10.45 a. m.

On June 21 500 c. c., representing the aqueous extract of 1,000 grams of the dried *Astragalus mollissimus*, were again fed. The animal now weighed 26.9 kilos. On June 26 the animal weighed 26 kilos, and its gait was very uncertain. The temperature was 104.2° F. It was fed 300 c. c. of fluid, representing the extract of 400 grams of the dried *Astragalus mollissimus*. On June 29 the animal weighed 26.8 kilos and the temperature was 102.8° F. It was fed the extract of 1,000 grams of dried *Astragalus mollissimus* in 500 c. c. of water. On June 30, at 10.45 a. m., the temperature was 104.2° F. The animal was very dull and died at night.

At autopsy the intestines and stomach merely appeared pale. There were no worms, and the lungs and other organs appeared normal.

Experiment No. 2.—A lamb weighing 15.4 kilos was fed on July 6, at 1.10 p. m., with 640 c. c. of fluid, representing the extract of 2,000 grams of *Astragalus mollissimus*. At 1.17 p. m. the animal could be turned on its back, and it regained its feet with difficulty. At 1.24 p. m. it urinated and had a stool. The lamb died during the night.

The autopsy the following morning showed the heart filled with clots; lungs normal save for hypostatic congestion. The cerebral and dural vessels were dilated. About 1½ teaspoonfuls of bloody serum were found at the base of the brain. There was none in the lateral ventricles, and no clots. The kidneys exhibited no marked congestion. There was no fluid found in the peritoneal or the pleural or pericardial cavities. The first stomach, however, contained small hemorrhagic spots, and the second was black. There were small hemorrhages in the intestines.

Experiment No. 3.—July 13, 1906, a sheep weighing 19.5 kilos was fed with 640 c. c. of fluid, representing the extract of 2,000 grams of *Aragallus lamberti*. The temperature at the time of feeding, 1.10 p. m., was 105.3° F. At 1.49 p. m. the sheep could be easily turned on its back. At 2.23 p. m. the temperature was 103.6° F. At 3.42 p. m. the temperature was 103.5° F. At 4.20 p. m. the respiration was fairly rapid. On July 14, at 11.15 a. m., the temperature was 103.6° F. The sheep would run about but could easily be turned over. It had not eaten, but there was diarrhea present. July 15, at 3.30 p. m., the temperature was 104° F. The animal had eaten. On July 17 the temperature was 104° F. and the animal weighed 18.8 kilos. On the 27th it weighed 17.2 kilos; on August 29, 20.8 kilos.

Experiment No. 4.—A lamb weighing 19 kilos was fed August 21, 1906, with 740 c. c., representing the aqueous extract of 2,500 grams of the fresh *Astragalus mollissimus*, shipped to Washington in September, 1905. This animal ate at night, but the following day was dull. When seen on August 27 there was diarrhea present and the animal was still dull. On the 28th the animal died, weighing 16.7 kilos. There was no autopsy on account of decomposition.

Experiment No. 5.—A lamb weighing 15.6 kilos was fed on September 4, 1906, with an aqueous extract representing 3,500 grams of the dried *Aragallus lamberti*, 1,000 c. c. of water being used. The temperature at the time of feeding was 104.3° F. At 2.48 p. m. the animal on rising to its feet developed a slight tremor of the fore legs and showed marked disinclination to stand on its feet. The temperature was 104° F. The animal died at 4.25 p. m. The post-mortem was negative, save for some reddening of the second stomach.[a]

These feeding experiments in sheep can not be considered quantitative, because, as is shown later, aqueous extracts of dried plants are often inactive, yet poisonous principles may be obtained from the plants by treatment with digestive fluids.

Extracts of dried loco plants vary much in their toxicity; with some the writer was unable to kill rabbits, even when an extract of 300 grams of the dried plant was used. It is interesting to note that when the field station was established at Hugo, Colo., in 1905, almost all the aqueous extracts of dried specimens sent to Washington would produce the acute symptoms of poisoning in rabbits, but during the third season of its existence many of the samples sent from the same area were much less active, if not inactive.

LABORATORY EXPERIMENTS—CHEMICAL.

The fact that the aqueous extract of 500 grams of the fresh *Astragalus mollissimus*, or of 200 grams (in some cases 100 grams) of the dried plant, when fed by mouth, would regularly kill a rabbit weighing about 907 grams, with certain definite clinical symptoms and pathological lesions, was at first arbitrarily selected as our test

---

[a] There was a slight odor of chloroform noticed on opening the stomach, so that perhaps the imperfect removal of the chloroform due to a hurried evaporation of the extract should be taken into consideration in this case.

to aid in the isolation of the active principle. Later the production of chronic symptoms by the aqueous extract or digestion of 200 grams of these dried plants given in doses of 100 grams each on two successive days was considered essential. Carnivora, such as dogs and cats, vomit so easily as to render them unsuitable for these investigations. The aqueous extract was distilled with and without steam, also after acidifying with sulphuric acid, and likewise after the addition of magnesium oxid, but in all cases the distillate was inactive.

The concentrated aqueous extract was shaken by the Dragendorff method with petroleum ether, benzol, chloroform, ether, and amyl alcohol, both in alkaline and acid condition, but the shakings yielded no physiologically active body. Shakings by the Otto-Stas method also proved inactive. Lead acetate, lead subacetate, silver nitrate, mercuric chlorid, alcohol, phosphotungstic acid, trichloracetic acid, ammonium hydrate, sodium carbonate, sodium hydrate, Mayer's solution, uranyl acetate, silver oxid, and barium carbonate also failed to remove the active constituent. They gave heavy precipitates in all cases, but these proved inactive. Hydrocyanic acid was sought for with negative results. The pathological lesions in the very acute cases suggested in some respects oxalic acid, a saponin, a metal, or perhaps a toxalbumin as the active principle, but none of the precipitants for saponins, such as lead and copper, or the magnesium oxid method yielded a body which was active. Proteids were excluded by the fact that the various proteid precipitants—alcohol, trichloracetic acid, lead subacetate, mercuric sulphate or chlorid, and salting out with ammonium sulphate and sodium chlorid (complete saturation and half saturation)—failed to give an active precipitate. Glucosidal or alkaloidal bodies were also excluded. On dialysing for twenty-four hours, some of the active principle went into the dialysate and some remained in the dialyser. Ether yielded a precipitate from alcoholic solution which failed to kill. The possibility of the activity of the plants being due to its normal acidity was excluded by neutralizing the extract with sodium hydrate and precipitating the salts with alcohol. The filtrate proved active after removing the alcohol.

The negative results in looking for active alkaloidal, or glucosidal, or proteid bodies suggested that perhaps the action was due to some inorganic constituent. The writer then boiled the extract three minutes and as the filtrate was still found active and the proteid precipitate inactive became convinced of the inorganic nature of the active constituents, and finally incinerated the plant. The acid extract from this was also active, but death was delayed several hours. This was believed to be due to the insoluble form into which the compound was converted.[c] In fact, the question of solubility and the avoidance of an acid reaction, which of itself may kill, are the main points to keep in mind.

These experiments indicated that the injurious action toward rabbits of the *Astragalus mollissimus* and *Aragallus lamberti* collected at Hugo, Colo., was due to one or more inorganic constituents,[b] but it does not follow that all loco plants have the same poisonous principle nor that the same species occurring on all soils has the same poisonous action.[c]

Of *Astragalus mollissimus* from Imperial, Nebr., collected in 1906, 200 grams were ashed in a platinum bowl and extracted with water. This aqueous extract when neutralized produced no marked symptoms in a rabbit and the weight of the animal remained about the same.

The ash undissolved after this extraction was then treated with acetic acid and water overnight, and after carefully evaporating off the acetic acid on the bath (tested by litmus paper) the residue was fed, partly in solution and partly suspended in water, to a rabbit weighing 1,800.2 grams. Next day the rabbit weighed 1,771.8 grams, showed paralysis of the limbs, and died during the morning. The stomach was intensely reddened and contracted.

An extract of a similar ash was made by boiling the same amount with a large quantity of 94 per cent alcohol. This was evaporated in vacuo and taken in water and fed to a rabbit weighing 1,459.9 grams. On the sixth day the animal died, having lost 70.9 grams in weight. The stomach showed reddening but no ulcers.

An acetic acid aqueous extract, made from the ash after the alcoholic extraction, proved inactive, showing that the alcohol had re-

---

[a] Work is now being done by the writer on the inorganic constituents of various plants.

[b] Scattered throughout the veterinary literature one finds cases of poisoning in animals with symptoms similar to those occurring in locoed animals which are attributed to eating plants grown on a peculiar soil, as in Oserow, Ueber Krankh. d. Pferde, welche Aehnlichkeit mit der Cerebro-spinal meningitis haben, aber durch Vergiftungen mit Gräsern von Salzgründen (Salzmooren) verursacht werden, Journ. f. Allgem. Veterinär-Medicin, St. Petersburg. p. 486, 1906. Abstract in Jahresber. über d. Leistungen auf dem Gebiete d. Veterinär-Medicin, vol. 26, p. 226. 1906.—Compare also Étude sur Quelques Plantes Vénéneuses des Regions Calcaires, Bul. Soc. Cent. de Méd. Vét., vol. 48, p. 378. 1894.

[c] After completing this work the writer found that Sayre had said that he "had the suggestion that the harm coming from this plant is due to the inorganic constituents; this clue has been followed up, but like the others has brought us no nearer to the solution of the problem." Kans. Acad. Sci. Trans., vol. 18, p. 144. 1903.

moved the active bodies. A 70 per cent alcohol extract of another ashed lot proved active, killing the rabbit overnight.

Of *Astragalus mollissimus* from Imperial, Nebr., 200 grams were ashed in a platinum bowl and the ash treated with acetic acid water. After freeing from acid, one half of the solution and emulsion was fed one day and the second half fed the following day. The rabbit at the time of feeding weighed 1,275.7 grams. Fourteen days later the animal died, weighing 1,105.6 grams. No autopsy.

A similar extract of the ash from between 100 and 150 grams of the same dried plant produced death in a rabbit weighing 1,190 grams in two hours and fifty-eight minutes.

The acetic acid extract of the ash of 125 grams of a mixture of the dried *Astragalus mollissimus* and *Aragallus lamberti* received from Hugo, Colo., June, 1907, after freeing from acid, was fed to a rabbit weighing 1,304 grams on July 29. On July 30 it weighed 1,332.4 grams. August 1 it weighed 1,219 grams, and it died the same day. The stomach was reddened and showed ulcers.

A similar extract from 250 grams of the same dried plants on boiling gave a heavy precipitate, but this precipitate was inactive, while the filtrate killed a rabbit in four hours.

Of dry *Aragallus lamberti* collected in September, 1906, 200 grams were extracted with water and fed to a rabbit weighing 1,516.7 grams. Two days later the animal weighed 1,360 grams and died the same day.

The ash from 200 grams of the same dried plant was extracted with acetic acid, and after evaporating off the acid this was fed to a rabbit weighing 2,045.3 grams. Seven days later the animal weighed 1,729.3 grams, having lost 316 grams in weight.

The ash from 250 grams of the same species of plant, after similar treatment with acetic acid, induced death in a rabbit weighing 2,069 grams in 2 hours and 20 minutes. The stomach was inflamed.

EFFECT OF THE AQUEOUS EXTRACT OF ASHED LOCO PLANTS.

The filtrate from the ash from 200 grams of dried *Astragalus mollissimus*, from Imperial, Nebr., after similar treatment with acetic acid water and freed from free acid, killed a rabbit in several hours.

Hydrochloric acid also rendered the toxic agent of the ash soluble in water, but proved unsuitable for our work, as it was found impossible to obtain neutral residues by mere evaporation on the bath. At first one of the heavy metals or members of the H_2S group [a] was suspected, but on passing H_2S into the slightly acid extract of the ash no

---

[a] Swain, R. E., and Harkins, W. D. Arsenic in Vegetation Exposed to Smelter Smoke. Journ. Amer. Chem. Soc., vol. 30, p. 915. 1908.—Harkins, W. D., and Swain, R. E. The Chronic Arsenical Poisoning of Herbivorous Animals. Journ. Amer. Chem. Soc., vol. 30, p. 928, 1908.

active precipitate resulted, but the filtrate remained active.[a] A special Marsh test was, however, made for arsenic and antimony with negative results. A test for tungsten with zinc and hydrochloric acid proved negative.

Members of the ammonium sulphid group were then suspected, but while ammonium hydrate alone gave a heavy white precipitate, this precipitate, as also the black one with ammonium sulphid, proved inactive save when not thoroughly freed from acid (used for solution). The action of this ammonium sulphid precipitate on rabbits was watched for sixteen days, but without result. Nevertheless, the writer still suspected some of the rare earths.[b]

Sestini [c] had found that if certain plants were nourished with a solution of a beryllium salt, in the ash of these plants could be shown the presence of beryllium.

Two grams of beryllium chlorid were fed in aqueous solution to a rabbit weighing 1,800.2 grams. In four days this animal lost 241 grams and died. The stomach showed the same general pallor seen in chronic locoed rabbits, but no ulcers. The tests for beryllium by Sestini's method, however, failed to show beryllium in the active loco plants examined.

Thorium chlorid, cerium chlorid, and lanthanum chlorid in 2-gram doses and zirconium chlorid in 3-gram doses produced no chronic symptoms in rabbits or, in fact, any disturbance. Titanium chlorid, 2.5 grams, evaporated in the air and then fed in an emulsion to a rabbit, also proved inactive, but this inactivity may have been due to its insolubility.

Thallium nitrate c. p., in aqueous solution, in 2-gram doses, killed a rabbit weighing 2,154.6 grams in two hours and fifteen minutes. The stomach in this case, while pink, was not hemorrhagic.

Zirconium chlorid has an astringent taste, and if fed repeatedly will cause the metallic astringent action. On boiling an acetic acid solution of the ash with sodium acetate a precipitate formed.[d]

The presence of zirconium was thus suspected and Dr. E. C. Sullivan, of the United States Geological Survey, estimated it to be

---

[a] A similar extract was sent to the Bureau of Chemistry, and that Bureau also reported an absence of the elements of the H_2S group.

[b] Bachem, C. Pharmakologisches über einige Edelerden. Arch. Internat. de Pharmacodyn., vol. 17, p. 363. 1907.

[c] Sestini, F. Esper. di Vegetaz. del Frumento con Sostituz. della Glucina alla Magnesia. Staz. Sper. Agrar. Ital., vol. 20, p. 256. 1891.—Di alcuni Elementi Chimici Rari a Trovarsi nei Vegetabili. Staz. Sper. Agrar. Ital., vol. 15, p. 290. 1888.

NOTE.—The ammonium sulphid precipitate was very small if the phosphates were first removed with tin and nitric acid.

[d] Böhm, C. R. Darstellung d. seltenen Erden, vol. 1, p. 40. 1905.

present in the ash of a sample of *Aragallus lamberti* in about 0.01 per cent zirconium oxid, with also 0.1 per cent titanium dioxid.[a]

Zirconium chlorid, 3 grams, was fed in aqueous solution to a rabbit weighing 850.5 grams. This rabbit lost 96 grams in seven days, and was then fed 3 grams more of the same solution and the following day 2 grams more. It died eight days later, weighing 656 grams. The stomach and intestines were contracted, but showed no ulcers. However, 4 grams killed a rabbit in two hours and thirty-two minutes.

The filtrate, after treating an active solution of the ash with hydrogen peroxid, proved active, thus showing that zirconium was not entirely responsible for the poisonous action.

Yttrium, while not found in the plant, was administered as yttrium chlorid to a rabbit weighing 1,530 grams in 2-gram doses in solution. This animal gained 113.4 grams in five days.

Didymium chlorid c. p., in 3-gram doses, was fed to a rabbit weighing 1,020 grams. This rabbit lost 70 grams in four days.

The administration of manganese acetate[b] in 2-gram doses was followed by a gain in weight of a rabbit of 42.5 grams, while a dose of 3 grams killed a rabbit weighing 1,077 grams in two hours and thirty minutes. Wohlwill[c] has emphasized the fact that the members of the iron group owe their comparative harmlessness to not being absorbed by the gastro-intestinal tract.

No zinc was found in the plant.[d]

It is well recognized that potassium salts given hypodermically are decidedly toxic and that ammonium salts given per os will kill, so that the writer considered the possibility of other members of the group being responsible for the injurious action. The fact that the alkaline distillate of the plant proved inactive eliminated the ammonium salts.

Cæsium chlorid c. p., 2 grams, was fed in aqueous solution to a rabbit weighing 1,077.2 grams. In six days this animal lost 255 grams in weight, when it died.[e]

---

[a] Wait, C. E. Occurrence of Titanium. Journ. Amer. Chem. Soc., vol. 18, p. 402. 1896.

NOTE.—There seem to be no records of any study of the pharmacological action of titanium.

[b] Compare Jaksch, R. v. Ueber Mangantoxikosen und Manganophobie. Münch. Med. Woch., p. 969. 1907.

[c] Wohlwill, F. Ueber d. Wirkung d. Metalle d. Nickelgruppe. Arch. f. Exper. Path., vol. 56, p. 409. 1907.

[d] Laband, L. Zur Verbreitung des Zinkes im Pflanzenreiche. Zeits. f. Untersuch. d. Nahrungs- u. Genussmittel, vol. 4, p. 489. 1901.

[e] Cæsium occurs in various plants and the possibility of poisoning by this element must be considered. It is hoped that the writer may be able to undertake a more thorough pharmacological study of this element.

A second rabbit, weighing 1,020.5 grams, was fed with 2 grams of the same solution and lost 368 grams in twenty-one days. The spectroscopic test, however, failed to show cæsium in the ashed plant. Rubidum chlorid c. p., in 2-gram doses, proved inactive. The platinum chlorid precipitate from the extract of the plant proved inactive.

The fact that the filtrate after precipitation of the phosphates by tin and nitric acid and H_2S was active excluded the phosphoric acid radical, and the filtrate after treatment with $BaCO_3$ and AgO being active excluded the H_2SO_4 and HCl radicals as the toxic body. Fluorine was proved to be absent.

A radio-active substance was suspected, but Dr. L. J. Briggs, Physicist of Bureau of Plant Industry, reported that the dried plant showed no special amount of radio-activity.[a]

Power and Cambier, Sayre, and Kennedy had previously called attention to the abundance of calcium in the plant, and the writer's investigations confirm this. Pharmacologists are averse to believing calcium given per os poisonous. The writer has, however, fed 5 grams of the acetate of calcium in solution to a rabbit weighing 652 grams. This animal died in two hours, with marked irritation of the stomach, the result being due to the so-called "salt action." Much larger amounts were fed in divided doses, but without injury. Calcium phosphate and calcium sulphate in 2-gram doses proved harmless to a rabbit weighing about 1,400 grams. Three grams of magnesium acetate [b] were fed in solution for five successive days to a rabbit weighing 1,417 grams, but without apparent effect.

Strontium acetate c. p., in 2-gram doses, likewise caused no disturbance.[c] No strontium in any amount recognizable by chemical tests was proved in the plant. So that by a process of exclusion the writer was forced to think of barium as the main cause of the trouble.

The writer noted that if the ashed plant was extracted with H_2SO_4 water and this extract freed from sulphuric acid with $PbCO_3$ and H_2S the solution proved inactive to rabbits and also that after this extraction the acetic acid extract of the ash failed to kill. In other words, the sulphate of our body was insoluble in water. At times in passing H_2S into active solutions of the ashed plant freed from the acetic acid by evaporation the filtrate and likewise the precipi-

---

[a] Acqua, C. Sull'accumulo di Sostanze Radioattive nei Vegetali. Atti della Reale Accad. dei Lincei, 5 s, vol. 16, sem. 2, p. 357. 1907.

[b] Compare Meltzer, S. J. Toxicity of Magnesium Nitrate When Given by Mouth. Science, vol. 26, p. 473. 1907.

[c] Burgassi, G. Modificaz. del Ricambio per Azione dello Stronzio. Archiv. di Farmacol., vol. 6, p. 551. 1907.

tate were inactive. Noyes and Bray [a] have noted that if H_2S is passed into certain solutions in the presence of an oxydizing agent, such as ferric iron, H_2SO_4 would be formed, which would throw any barium out of solution.

In one blood-pressure record made with a dog (vagi nerves cut), a rise in blood pressure (a characteristic physiological action of barium) was seen to follow the intravenous injection of the aqueous extract of the plant, in spite of its normal acid reaction.

Accidentally the writer found that Sprengel [b] had reported the presence of barium in *Astragalus exscapus*, a closely allied plant. Barium has also been found in the vegetable world by Scheele in 1788, and later by Eckard,[c] who found it in beeoh, while Forchhammer [d] proved it in birch, and Lutterkorth found it in the soil of the same area in which Eckard worked. Dworzak [e] noted the occurrence of traces of this element in wheat grown along the Nile, and Knop [f] found it in the soil. Doctor Balfour, of Khartum, Egypt, informed the writer that he knew of no cases in which this barium in wheat had produced poisoning. Hornberger [g] found barium both in the red beech grown in Germany and in the soil on which these trees grew. It has also been claimed that various marine plants may take up barium from the sea.[h]

---

[a] Noyes, A. A., and Bray, W. C. System of Qualitative Analysis for the Common Elements. Journ. Amer. Chem. Soc., vol. 29, pp. 168, 172, and 191. 1907.

NOTE.—Barium sulphate is nontoxic on account of its insolubility. Orfila fed 16–24 grams to dogs without causing any disturbance. Bary, A. Beitr. z. Baryumwirkung. Dorpat, 1888, p. 25.

[b] Sprengel, C. Von den Substanzen der Ackerbrume und des Untergrundes, Journ. f. Techn. u. Œkon. Chem., vol. 3, p. 313. 1828.

[c] Eckard, G. E. Baryt, ein Bestandtheil der Asche des Buchenholzes. Annal. der Chem. u. Pharm., n. s., vol. 23, p. 294. 1856.

[d] Forchhammer, J. G. Ueber den Einfluss des Kochsalzes auf die Bildung der Mineralien. Annal. d. Physik u. Chemie, vol. 5, p. 91. 1905.—Lutterkorth, H. Kohlensäurer Baryt, ein Bestandtheil des Sandsteines in der Gegend von Göttingen. Annal. d. Chem. u. Pharm., n. s., vol. 23, p. 296. 1856.

[e] Dworzak, H. Baryt unter den Aschenbestandtheilen des Ægyptischen Weizen. Landw. Versuchs.-Stat., vol. 17, p. 398. 1874.

[f] Knop, W. Analysen von Nilabsatz. Landw. Versuchs.-Stat., vol. 17, p. 65. 1874.—Compare also Demoussy, E., Absorption par les Plantes de Quelques Sels Solubles, Thése, Paris, 1899.—Knop, W., Einige neue Resultate der Untersuchung über die Ernährung der Pflanze, Ber. ü. Verhandl. d. königl. sächs. Gesells. d. Wissens. zu Leipzig, Math. Phys. Cl., vol. 29, p. 113, 1877.—Suzuki, U., Can Strontium and Barium Replace Calcium in Phænogams? Bul. Coll. Agric. Tokio Imp. Univ., vol. 4, p. 69, 1900–1902.

[g] Hornberger, R. Ueber d. Vorkommen d. Baryums in d. Pflanze und im Boden. Landw. Versuchs.-Stat., vol. 51, p. 473. 1899.

[h] Roscoe, H. E., and Schorlemmer, C. Treatise on Chemistry, vol. 2, p. 455. 1897.

Hillebrand [a] has called attention to the fact that the igneous rocks of the Rocky Mountains showed a higher percentage of barium than rock from other portions of the United States, so that under these conditions one might expect the presence of barium in plants growing in this region. A sample of *Aragallus lamberti* and one of *Astragalus mollissimus* were sent to the Bureau of Chemistry for spectroscopic examination for various elements and they reported traces of barium in each.[b]

With these arguments the writer felt sure of the presence of barium, and the matter was discussed with Dr. E. C. Sullivan, of the United States Geological Survey, and he kindly corroborated the conclusions reached as to the presence of barium, controlling its presence by means of the spectroscope, and estimated it roughly as 0.1 per cent BaO in the ash of a sample of *Aragallus lamberti* (6.3 milligrams $BaSO_4$ in 4 grams ash). This determination was made by Hillebrand's method.

Kobert has anticipated this result, saying that " all plants are in the position occasionally to take up barium combinations from the soil," and " the plants which thus contain barium may act injuriously to men and animals." [c]

TOTAL ASH DETERMINATIONS OF LOCO PLANTS.

The reports of the ash analyses of the loco plants show marked variations in the total amount of the ash. Thus, from *Aragallus lamberti* Dyrenforth obtained 4.32 per cent and O'Brine 13.52 per cent of ash. The Bureau of Chemistry analyzed two different samples of this dried plant and reported in one case 11.15 per cent and in the second 11.64 per cent of ash. O'Brine [d] obtained 13.52

---

[a] Hillebrand, W. F. Analysis of Silicate and Carbonate Rocks. Dept. Interior, U. S. Geol. Survey, Bul. 305, p. 18. 1907.

[b] This report came from the Plant Analysis Laboratory of the Bureau of Chemistry, a different one from that which later controlled the writer's tests quantitatively and qualitatively. In other words, the conclusions of the writer as to the presence of barium were controlled by three separate individuals.

[c] Kobert, R. Kann ein in einem Pflanzenpulver gefundener abnorm höher Barytgehalt erklärt werden durch direkte Aufnahme von Baryumsalze durch die lebende Pflanze aus dem Boden? Chem. Zeit., vol. 10, p. 491. 1899.

NOTE.—The writer has also found barium in entirely different botanical families from the loco weed, and it is hoped a report can shortly be made of some of these.

NOTE.—The first sample of ash analyzed by the Bureau of Chemistry had 0.21 per cent Fe_2O_3, 0.92 per cent Al_2O_3, 0.98 per cent CaO, 0.37 per cent MgO, 5.50 per cent SiO_2. The second lot was only examined for certain constituents, and gave K_2O, 2.25 per cent; CaO, 1.20 per cent; MgO, 0.41 per cent; P_2O_5, 0.52 per cent; and SO_3, 0.24 per cent.

[d] The detailed analysis of O'Brine can be found on page 32 of this report.

129

per cent of ash from the same species. The writer's analysis [a] gave in one sample of *Aragallus lamberti*, collected at Hugo, Colo., in 1907, 18.8 per cent of ash; a second lot (1907), 12.44 per cent; a third (1906), 11 per cent, and a fourth (May, 1905) gave 37.3 per cent of ash.[b] One lot from Woodland Park, Colo. (October, 1906), gave 6.4 per cent. One lot from Hugo, Colo. (October, 1907), yielded 9.6 per cent.

In the case of *Astragalus mollissimus*, Wentz obtained 6.76 per cent, Sayre 12.01 per cent, Kennedy 20 per cent, O'Brine 12.15 per cent, while the sample analyzed by the Bureau of Chemistry gave 18.4 per cent of ash. One sample from Kit Carson County, Colo. (December, 1906), which proved inactive physiologically, gave an ash content of 6.9 per cent. A sample of *Astragalus missouriensis* collected at Hugo, Colo., June, 1907, yielded an ash content of 21.8 per cent, and an *Astragalus missouriensis* collected at Pierre, S. Dak., September, 1907, yielded 27 per cent. An *Astragalus nitidus* from Custer, S. Dak. (July, 1907), gave 5.2 per cent ash, while an *Astragalus nitidus* collected at Woodland Park, Colo., in October, 1906, yielded 7.8 per cent, and another specimen of *Astragalus nitidus* also collected at Woodland Park, Colo., in October, 1907, gave 12.2 per cent. An *Astragalus drummondii* from Custer, S. Dak. (July, 1907), gave 5.9 per cent. *Astragalus pectinatus* (Hugo, June, 1907) yielded 6.1 per cent. A fresh (undried) specimen of *Astragalus mollissimus* (unknown origin, November, 1907) yielded 3.8 per cent of ash. One sample of *Astragalus decumbens* (Ephraim, Utah, August, 1907) gave 21.8 per cent of ash.

These determinations must necessarily be only approximate, as the plants were collected by different persons who exercised different degrees of care in freeing them from adherent soil, and possibly in drying the plants, so that the main value of these figures is their aid in determining the amount of barium present.

BARIUM DETERMINATIONS IN THE ASH OF LOCO PLANTS.

Attention has been called to the fact that in ashing plants containing barium a part at least of this barium is converted into the insoluble sulphate and a part into the carbonate, so that the characteristic pharmacological action of the ash will depend not upon the total barium present, but upon the form in which it occurs— little action if much $BaSO_4$ and more complete if more $BaCO_3$ results. A further difficulty in the recognition of barium in plants

---

[a] All ash and barium determinations were made from the dried plants save when otherwise specified.

[b] Evidently these plants must have been imperfectly freed from soil.

is due to the fact that certain inorganic salts interfere with the precipitation by H_2SO_4.

A specimen of *Aragallus lamberti* (Hugo, summer of 1907) with 12.44 per cent of ash was examined for its barium content by Hillebrand's method.[a] The method was as follows:

Two grams of the ash were first fused with sodium carbonate and the fused mass washed with water containing sodium carbonate. The residue was washed into a beaker and treated with a few drops of sulphuric acid. The residue now remaining was filtered and after ignition was treated with hydrofluoric and sulphuric acids. After evaporating off these acids, the residue was treated with sulphuric acid water, filtered, and then fused with sodium carbonate. After extracting with sodium carbonate water, the residue was dissolved in just enough hydrochloric acid and precipitated with sulphuric acid. The precipitate was dissolved in concentrated sulphuric acid and reprecipitated by water and weighed as $BaSO_4$.[b] So far as the writer can ascertain, there have been no control experiments made for this method to determine the experimental error.

Of the above ash, 1.998 grams gave 5.2 milligrams of $BaSO_4$, which would correspond to 75.75 milligrams of barium acetate crystals—$Ba(C_2H_3O_2)_2 + H_2O$—in 200 grams of the dried plant. The residue by the Hillebrand method after weighing was tested with the spectroscope and gave a bright spectrum for barium. The same ash was analyzed by the Bureau of Chemistry, using a shorter method, and they reported 2.7 milligrams of barium sulphate in 1.1217 grams of ash. A second sample collected earlier in the summer, with an ash content of 18.6 per cent, was shown to yield barium corresponding to 3.4 milligrams of $BaSO_4$ in 2.5 grams of the ash.[c]

One lot of *Aragallus lamberti* collected at Hugo, Colo., in May, 1905, and which gave an ash content of 37.3 per cent, was found to yield 3 milligrams of $BaSO_4$ from 1.998 grams of ash, or 173.88 milligrams of $Ba(C_2H_3O_2)_2 + H_2O$ in 200 grams of the dried plant, but this ash also contained 0.27 per cent of SO_3. The Bureau of Chemistry reported the barium to correspond to 2.9 milligrams of $BaSO_4$ in 2.45 grams of the ash.

The *Astragalus missouriensis* (Hugo, June, 1907), with an ash content of 21.8 per cent, gave 3 milligrams of $BaSO_4$ in 2.01 grams

---

[a] Hillebrand, W. F. Analysis of Silicate and Carbonate Rocks. U. S. Geol. Surv. Bul. 305, p. 116. 1907. See also Folin, O., On the Reduction of Barium Sulphate in Ordinary Gravimetric Determinations, in Journ. Biol. Chem., vol. 3, p. 81. 1907.

[b] All the determinations of barium which resulted either positively or negatively were made with the same bottle of sodium carbonate and H_2SO_4, so that impurities in the chemicals were thus eliminated.

[c] Report from Bureau of Chemistry.

of ash, or 76.58 milligrams of $Ba(C_2H_3O_2)_2+H_2O$ in 200 grams of the dried plant. The residue after weighing was tested spectroscopically and gave a bright barium spectrum.

The *Astragalus drummondii* from Custer, S. Dak. (1906), *Astragalus mollissimus* from Kit Carson County, Colo. (December, 1906), and *Astragalus nitidus* from Woodland Park, Colo. (October, 1907), were reported by the Bureau of Chemistry to contain no barium.

The ash of the *Astragalus pectinatus* (Hugo, June, 1907) was reported by the Bureau of Chemistry to show no barium on spectroscopic examination.

Two grams of active loco plant ash yielded from 5 to 6 milligrams of $BaSO_4$, but it can be easily seen that in multiplying this amount to correspond to 200 grams of the dried plant errors would be likely to arise, so that the whole amount of barium would not necessarily be accounted for.

ANALYSIS OF SOILS.

One sample of the soil from near Hugo, Colo., from which the *Aragallus lamberti* was collected, was examined by the Bureau of Soils, and that Bureau reported the absence of barium and zirconium, at least of any recognizable by the chemical methods used, so that it can not be said that the barium came from any soil accidentally mixed with the ash. Traces of titanium were, however, found. Evidently the plant must collect minimal quantities of these elements from the soil and store them.

The water from a well of an adjacent area was examined by the Bureau of Chemistry and reported to contain 37.4 parts of calcium and 13.7 parts of magnesium in one million, and that the water contained no barium.[a]

FEEDING EXPERIMENTS WITH BARIUM SALTS ON ANIMALS IN THE LABORATORY.

On these figures the writer took 0.2 gram of crystallized barium acetate c. p., using the acetate because acetic acid has been proved in certain loco plants by Power and Cambier, and after dissolving it in water fed it at 9.45 a. m. to a rabbit weighing 1,177 grams. The head soon fell forward so that the nose rested on the ground. At 10.58 a. m. the rabbit seemed unable to guide itself and would run into obstructions if forced to move. There was no diarrhea but it urinated several times. There was a peculiar tremor of the muscles noted. The animal would not startle by sudden noises and at 11.06

---

[a] Barium has been found in well water in England. See Thorpe, T. E., Contribution to the History of the Old Sulphur Well, Harrogate, in Philos. Mag., 5 s., vol. 2, p. 50, 1876.

a. m. could be placed on its back with ease. The pupils appeared about normal. The whites of the eyes showed very prominently. At 11.35 a. m. the fore legs were paralyzed. The following morning the animal was dead, its weight being 1.120 grams. The heart was dilated; the stomach was not hemorrhagic, but rather pale.

A second rabbit, which weighed 1.680 grams, was fed with a solution of 0.5 gram of the same salt at 9.42 a. m. At 10.35 a. m. the animal passed soft stools and showed a marked disinclination to move, with evidence of pain. The diarrhea [a] became more marked and the animal's hind quarters were soiled with feces. At 10.48 a. m. there was marked incoordination of the limbs and inability to stand. Finally, at 10.56 a. m., convulsions began and the animal died at 11.02 a. m. The autopsy was made about two hours later. The animal was then rigid. The kidneys seemed rather congested. The intestines were relaxed; mesenteric vessels dilated. The pyloric region of the stomach appeared hemorrhagic.

A third rabbit, fed like the preceding with 0.5 gram of barium acetate, showed much the same result. In this case there was some retching, but the other symptoms were as above, the animal dying in one hour and five minutes. No hemorrhages were seen in the stomach walls. It was noted that after the administration of certain doses, 0.2 gram, there was no diarrhea.

On September 23, 1907, a rabbit weighing 1.757 grams was fed at 10.42 a. m. with 0.1 gram of the same barium acetate. The temperature at the time of feeding was $102.9°$ F. At 12.05 a. m. the animal urinated. Temperature, $101.4°$ F. On September 24 the animal weighed the same. Temperature at 10.55 a. m., $102.3°$ F. The same amount of barium was fed. At 3.40 p. m. the temperature was $102.5°$ F. On September 25 the animal weighed 1,800 grams. Temperature, $102.2°$ F. at 10.39 a. m. The dose of barium was repeated. At 3.55 p. m. the temperature was $101.4°$ F. On September 26 at 9.38 a. m. the temperature was $101.1°$ F., and again the barium was given. At 3.57 p. m. the temperature was $101.5°$ F. On September

---

[a] Magnus, R. Wirkungsweise u. Angriffspunkt einiger Gifte am Katzendarm. Archiv. f. Gesam. Physiol., vol. 108. p. 44. 1905.

Note.—Reports on the histological changes in acute barium poisoning can be found in Pilliet. A. and Malbec. A. Note sur les Lesions Histologiques du Rein Produits par les Sels de Baryte sur les Animaux. Comp. Rend. Hebd. Soc. de Biol., vol. 4. p. 957. 1892.

Literature on the pharmacology of barium not otherwise referred to is as follows: Boehm. R. Ueber d. Wirkungen d. Barytsalze auf d. Thierkörper. Arch. f. Exp. Path., vol. 3. p. 217. 1875.—Sommer, F. Beitr. z. Kennt. d. Baryum-Vergiftung. Dissert., Würzburg. 1890.—Neumann. J. Ueber den Verbleib der in den thierischen Organismus eingeführten Bariumsalzen. Archiv. f. Gesam. Physiol., vol. 36, p. 576. 1885.—Heffter, A. Ausscheidung körperfremder Substanzen im Harn. Ergeh. d. Physiol., pt. 1, p. 121. 1903.—

27 the rabbit weighed 1,772 grams. The temperature at 9.53 a. m. was 102.3° F. The barium was fed for the fifth time. At 10.27 a. m. there were general convulsions. The eyes teared. At 10.32 a. m. soft stools appeared and the animal urinated. Stools were passed at various periods. At 11.30 a. m. there were no signs of pain on pinching the ear. At 11.58 a. m. the animal retched. The animal was lying with the fore legs wide apart and could not support itself. At 12.05· p. m. the temperature was 98° F. and the rabbit died shortly after.

The peritoneal cavity seemed normal. The small intestines were relaxed, while the mesenteric vessels were dilated. The kidneys seemed congested. The stomach walls were pink and in places covered with mucus. The heart was relaxed save the left ventricle, which seemed firm.

On September 23, 1907, a second rabbit, weighing 1,360 grams, was fed with a similar solution and the feeding was repeated at the same time the first rabbit was fed. On September 27 the animal weighed 1,416 grams. On this day a peculiar movement of the hind legs on jumping appeared, apparently due to an inability to draw the legs completely up, and the fore legs were spread wide apart, as if too weak to support the animal. The temperature had also fallen. On September 28 the animal had apparently recovered. Weight, 1,516 grams on October 21.

On September 23, 1907, a third rabbit, weighing 1,304 grams, was fed with 50 milligrams of barium acetate. This dose was repeated each time the other two rabbits were fed. On September 27 it weighed 1,304 grams. Marked muscular twitching appeared, with disinclination to move. Finally there were convulsions and paralysis of the limbs. No stools were seen. This animal lay quiet all night,

Binet, P. Recherches Compar. sur l'Action Physiol. des Métaux Alcalins et Alcalino-terreux. Rev. Méd. de la Suisse. Romande, vol. 12, pp. 535, 607. 1892.—Cyon, M. Ueber d. toxisch. Wirkung. d. Baryt- u. Oxalsäureverbindungen. Archiv. f. Anat., Physiol. u. Wissens. Med., 1866, p. 196.—Mickwitz, L. Vergleich. Untersuch. ü. d. physiol. Wirkung d. Salze d. Alcalien u. Alcal. Erden. Dissert., Dorpat, 1874.—Heilborn, F. Ueber Veränderungen im Darme nach Vergift. mit Arsen, Chlorbarium und Phosphor. Dissert., Würzburg, 1891.—Reincke, J. J. Ein Fall mehrfacher Vergiftung durch kohlensäuren Baryt. Viertelj. f. gerichtl. Med., n. s., vol. 28, p. 248. 1878.—Orfila, Mémoire sur l'Empoisonnement par les Alcalis Fixes. Journ. de Chimie Méd., 2 s., vol. 8. p. 200. 1842.—Santi, L. Se nel Veneficio per Sali di Bario questo Metallo passa alla Urina? Gazz. Chem. Ital., vol. 33, pt. 2, p. 202. 1903.—Weber, F. R. Barium Chloride. Milwaukee Med. Journ., vol. 12, pp. 39, 60. 1904.— Rabuteau. De l'Innocuité des Sels de Strontium Comparée a l'Activité du Chlorure de Baryum. Gaz. Méd. de Paris, 3 s., vol. 24, p. 218. 1869.—The very early literature is considered in detail by Bary.

apparently unable to move, and continued on its side until 3.15 p. m. on September 28, when it gradually recovered, weighing 1,346 grams on October 24.

On October 24, 1907, a rabbit weighing 1,346.5 grams was fed with a solution of 25 milligrams of crystallized barium acetate. On the next day the weight was 1,318 grams, and the dose was repeated. On October 26 it weighed 1,275.7 grams, and the dose was repeated; on October 30 it weighed 1,332 grams, and on October 31 its weight was 1,375 grams. The animal died at night on November 6; weight, 1,134 grams. The post-mortem examination, made with Dr. Meade Bolton, of the Bureau of Animal Industry, was negative save for the presence of necrotic tissue in one enlarged thyroid.

On October 24, 1907, a rabbit weighing 1,332 grams was fed with a solution of 25 milligrams of crystallized barium acetate. On the next day the animal weighed the same, and the dose was repeated. On October 26 it weighed 1,289 grams, and the same amount of barium was given. On October 28 the weight was 1,219 grams and two days later 1,289 grams.

On October 31, 1907, a rabbit weighing 723 grams was fed with a solution of 25 milligrams of barium acetate. This rabbit was fed in all nine times during a period of ten days. At the end of this time it weighed 779 grams and died six days later, weighing 723 grams. The post-mortem was negative.

A rabbit weighing 779 grams was also fed on October 31, 1907, with a similar amount of barium. This dose was repeated six times during an interval of eight days. At the end of that time the animal still retained its normal weight. On November 14, 1907, it weighed 709 grams, having lost 70 grams. Thus after daily doses of 0.1 gram of crystallized barium acetate no symptoms appeared until the fifth day, when death resulted. After the similar administration of 50 milligrams severe symptoms developed on the same day, but the animal recovered. After the administration of 25 milligrams on three successive days the animal died. In other cases of feeding 25 milligrams for several successive days, some lost weight and died; others merely lost in weight, but recovered.

Bary fed a rabbit weighing 0.9 kilogram a solution of 30 milligrams of barium chlorid on one day, on the second day 90 milligrams, and on the third day 30 milligrams. The only symptom noted was diarrhea. The animal died on the fifth day. In other words, after feeding small doses of barium salts for several days acute symptoms suddenly set in, showing a cumulative action. This cumulative action has been noted on man.[a]

---

[a] Bary, A. Beitr. z. Baryumwirkung. Dissert., Dorpat, 1888, p. 100.

Ousum [a] fed a medium-sized rabbit daily with small doses of barium carbonate, beginning with 20 milligrams. When the total amount reached 0.19 grams the rabbit died. The animal before death showed paralysis, respiratory disturbances, and fall in temperature. The sensibility of the cornea diminished, but the pupils responded to light. The stomach walls showed ecchymoses and the blood vessels of the brain, the spinal cord, and the abdominal vessels were dilated. Emboli in the pulmonary arteries were also noted.

In a rabbit the application of 0.66 gram of barium chlorid to a wound was followed in twenty minutes by convulsions, paralysis, and finally coma and death.[b]

Of barium nitrate 0.66 gram mixed with sugar and fed to a rabbit caused death in less than one hour, and 0.33 gram induced death in another rabbit in twenty-seven hours.[c]

Six grains (0.4 gram) of barium iodid fed in solution to a rabbit caused death the following day. On this day there were tremors of the neck and shoulders with convulsive movements of the limbs. There was also grinding of the teeth. " The mucous membrane of the stomach was rose-red at the cardia, and softened." Membranes of the cord and brain also were congested.[d]

For rabbits weighing 1,500 to 2,000 grams the lethal dose of barium chlorid on subcutaneous use is stated to be 0.05 to 0.06 grams.[e]

A rabbit weighing 1,106 grams was fed with a solution containing 50 milligrams of crystallized barium acetate c. p. and 50 milligrams of zirconium chlorid (pure). In fifty-seven minutes the animal showed difficulty in moving the fore legs, developing marked paralysis of the same about five hours later, and died the following morning—that is, twenty-two hours after feeding. The heart was found dilated, kidneys congested, stomach walls pink and covered in places with mucus and partly digested blood, and cerebral dural vessels dilated, but no clots were seen; bladder full.

Mixtures of 0.5 gram of calcium acetate and 50 milligrams of barium acetate failed to kill. Mixtures of titanium and barium were not tried, as no titanium salt soluble in water and of neutral reaction was accessible.

---

[a] Onsum, J. Ueber d. toxisch. Wirkung. der Baryt- und Oxalsäureverbindungen. Arch. f. Path. Anat., vol. 28, p. 234. 1863.

[b] Brodie, B. C. Further Experiments and Observations on the Action of Poisons on the Animal System. Philos. Trans., vol. 102, p. 218. 1812.

[c] Tidy, C. M. On Poisoning by Nitrate of Baryta. Med. Press and Circ., vol. 6, p. 448. 1868.

[d] Glover, R. M. On the Physiological and Medicinal Properties of Bromine and Its Compounds. Edinb. Med. & Surg. Journ., vol. 58, p. 341. 1842.

[e] Kissner, G. Ueber Baryum Vergiftungen u. deren Einfluss auf d. Glykogengehalt der Leber. Scholten, 1896, p. 11.

Mittelstaedt called attention to the fact that pregnant rabbits were more easily affected by the barium administration than nonpregnant ones, and noted abortion in one case.[a] One gram of the barium carbonate killed a dog in eight hours. A second dog died in fifteen hours. Both of these animals vomited so that a portion of this must have been lost.[b] Barium carbonate was formerly employed as a rat poison.[c]

Of barium chlorid 0.6 gram, fed in aqueous solution, caused death in a dog in forty-eight minutes if vomiting was prevented.[d]

In Tidy's hands 2 grams of the barium nitrate caused death in a small terrier in three and three-fourth hours. This dog had slight convulsions, was almost unable to stand, and had vomiting and purging. The reflexes were diminished. A small dog recovered only completely in five days after being fed 0.66 gram, while a large dog after being fed 1.3 grams only recovered after two days.

In cats 0.8 gram of barium carbonate when introduced into a wound caused on the third day languor, slow respiration, feeble pulse, twitching of hind legs, dilated pupils, and death.[e]

BARIUM POISONING IN MAN.

The high toxicity of barium was called attention to by early observers, but it was attributed by some to admixed arsenic. The reports of feeding experiments with barium on animals have varied markedly, but now care is being advised in the use of barium salts.[f]

Barium was introduced into medicine in the treatment of scrofula, but has fallen into disuse, and only recently attention has been called to it on account of its action on the circulatory system. Filippi,[g]

---

[a] Mittelstaedt, F. Ueber chronische Bariumvergiftung. Dissert., Greifswald, 1895, p. 19.

[b] Pelletier, D. Observations sur la Strontiane. Annal. de Chimie, vol. 21, p. 119. 1797.

[c] Christison, R. Treatise on Poisons. Edinburgh, 1845, p. 579.—Crampe, Bewährte Mittel gegen Feldmäuse. Deutsch. Landw. Presse, vol. 5, p. 530. 1878.—Felletar, E. Fälle von Intox. mit kohlensäur. Baryum. Pest. Med.-Chir. Presse, vol. 28, p. 1072. 1892.

[d] Husemann, T. Ein Beitrag z. Kennt. d. Barytvergiftungen. Zeits. f. pract. Heilk., vol. 3, p. 235. 1866. In this article Husemann has collected many cases of poisoning by barium in animals.

[e] Christison, R. Treatise on Poisons. Edinburgh, 1845, p. 579.

[f] According to v. Jaksch, " Sie ist bei der grossen Toxicität der Substanz immer ernst zu stellen." Vergiftungen, 1897, p. 79.

NOTE.—A thorough pharmacological study of some barium salt is much needed, and it is hoped that the writer will be able to complete this work.

[g] Filippi, E. Modificaz. del Ricambio Organice per Azione del Cloruro di Bario. La Sperimentale, vol. 60, p. 610. 1906; Sull' Azione Cardiaca del Chloruro di Bario. Archivio di Farmacol. Speriment., vol. 5, p. 122. 1906.

however, says, " The effects on the heart and on the pressure are already the first indication of poisoning." This metal has also been used in the treatment of chronic diseases of the spinal cord, as multiple sclerosis and paralysis agitans.[a]

After the administration to a woman of $\frac{1}{12}$ grain (0.005 gram) of barium chlorid three to five times a day for a few days, a total of $2\frac{1}{4}$ grains (0.135 gram), the patient developed rapid respiration, tenderness over the epigastrium, nausea, constipation, cramps in the limbs, loss of appetite, weakness, great emaciation, dysuria, some deafness with tinnitus, difficulty in speaking and thinking, with vertigo.[b] In this case the eyes were glassy, the vision indistinct, and the cheeks flushed. Kohl after the use of small doses of the same noted salivation, swelling of the gums, and falling out of the teeth, with a mercurial odor to the breath. Christison[c] states: " I have known violent vomiting, gripes, and diarrhea produced in like manner by a quantity not exceeding the usual medicinal doses." According to Kennedy few persons are able to bear $\frac{1}{8}$ grain (0.0075 gram) of barium chlorid.[d]

In Carpenter's case after three doses of 1.6 grains (0.070 gram) of barium chlorid the patient developed almost lethal symptoms.[e] Carpenter calls attention to the drowsiness which developed in this patient after the administration of barium, a fact which had already been noted by Christison.[f]

A cartarrhal affection of various mucous membranes and a swelling of various glands have been noted, especially of the lymph and salivary glands, and in the male the testes have at times swollen.[g] The inflammation of the glands may pass on to suppuration. The skin becomes dry and shows a tendency to crack. Febrile attacks are reported after the repeated use of small doses of barium.

---

[a] Schulz, H. Vorles. ü. Wirkung. u. Anwendung d. unorganisch. Arzneistoffe. Leipzig, 1907, p. 234.—Hare, H. A. Use of Barium Chloride in Heart Disease. Med. News, vol. 54, p. 183. 1889.

[b] Ferguson, J. C. Symptoms of Poisoning from Muriate of Barytes. Dublin Quart. Journ. Med. Sci., vol. 1, p. 271. 1846.

[c] Christison, R., l. c., p. 580.

[d] Kennedy, H. Dose of the Muriate of Barytes. Lancet, vol. 2, p. 28. 1873.

[e] Carpenter, J. S. Barium Chloride from a Clinical Standpoint. Med. News, vol. 59, p. 93. 1891.

[f] Christison, R., 1. c., 1845, p. 578.

[g] Schulz, H. Vorles. ü. Wirkung. u. Anwendung d. unorganisch. Arzneistoffe. Leipzig, 1907, p. 233.—Schwilgué, C. J. A. Traité de Mat. Méd., 3 ed., vol. 1, p. 441. 1818.

NOTE.—According to the files of the Office of Poisonous-Plant Investigations, E. D. Smith reported in the Orange Judd Farmer, 1897, that locoed animals showed a swelling of various glands. As yet the writer has been unable to verify this reference.

Scheibler [a] has called attention to the possibility of producing *chronic* barium poisoning in man from the use of barium in the manufacture of food products.

Acute cases of poisoning in man from four or more grams of barium carbonate or chlorid or nitrate have been reported more or less frequently.[b] In the acute case of poisoning in man reported by Tiraboschi and Taito, no macroscopic changes were noted in the stomach mucosa.[c] Lopes [d] has reported one case of acute poisoning in man from less than 1 gram of barium chlorid. In this case paralysis of the limbs was a marked feature. Stern [e] cites Perondi and Lisfranc to the effect that " remarkably large doses of barium chlorid can be borne without injury by gradually increasing the doses (dissolved in much water)." Lisfranc [f] has suggested that the sensitiveness to poisoning by barium salts is greater in certain climates than in others.

No data are as yet available as to the influence of altitude and partial starvation on the toxicity of barium salts. As is well known,

---

[a] Scheibler, C. Ueber d. Verwendung giftiger Stoffe, besonders d. Barytverbindungen bei d. Zuckerfabrication. Chem. Zeit., vol. 11, p. 1463. 1887.

[b] Schmidt's Jahrbücher, vol. 192, p. 131. 1881.—Walsh, J. Report of a Case of Poisoning by Chloride of Barium. Lancet, vol. 1, p. 211. 1859.—Walch. Seltener Fall einer tödlich. Vergiftung d. Baryta muriatica. Zeits. f. Staatsarznk., vol. 30, p. 1. 1835.—Carpenter, J. S. Barium Chloride from a Clinical Standpoint. Med. News, vol. 59, p. 93. 1891.—Eschricht. Dødeligt forløbende Forgiftning med salpetersurt Baryt. Ugeskrift for Laeger, vol. 4, p. 241. 1881.—Ogier and Socquet. Empoisonnement par le Chlorure de Baryum. Annal. d'Hyg. Publ., 3 s., vol. 25, p. 447. 1891.—Chevallier, A. Note sur un Cas d'Empoisonnement Déterminé par l'Acétate de Baryte. Annal. d'Hyg. Publ., 2 s., vol. 39, p. 395. 1873.—Courtin, Cas d'Empoisonnement par du Chlorure de Baryum. Rev. d'Hyg., vol. 4, p. 653. 1882.—Poisoning by a Baryta Compound. Pharm. Journ., 3 s., vol. 2, p. 1021. 1872.—Reichardt, E. Vergiftungsfall mit kohlensäurem Baryt. Arch. d. Pharm., 3 s., vol. 4, p. 426. 1874.—Lagarde, P. Acétate de Baryte livré sous le Nom de Sulfovinate de Soude. Union Méd., 3 s., vol. 14, p. 537. 1872.—Baum. Zwei Fälle von fahrlässiger Tödtung durch saltpetersäures Baryt. Zeits. f. Medizinalbeamte, vol. 9, p. 759. 1896.—Funaro, A. Sul Veneficio per Sali di Bario. L'Orosi, vol. 12, p. 397. 1894.

[c] Tiraboschi, A., and Taito, F. Avvelenamento da Bario. Il Risveglio Medico d'Abruzzo e Molise, vol. 1, p. 171. 1906.

NOTE.—A criticism of this case is to be found in Bellisari, G., Su Di un Presunto Avvelenamento da Bario. Il Risveglio Medico d'Abbruzzo e Molise, vol. 2, p. 15. 1907.

[d] Lopes, A. Caso Curioso de Envenenamento Pelo Chloret de Bario. Medicina Contempt., Lisbon, vol. 4, p. 109. 1886.

[e] Stern, E. Vergiftung mit Chlorbarium. Zeits. f. Medizinalbeamte, vol. 9, p. 383. 1896.

NOTE.—The writer has always theoretically questioned the danger of poisoning by loco weeds in well-fed and well-watered animals. Compare Stalker, M., The " Loco " Plant and Its Effect on Animals. Bur. Animal Industry, 3d Ann. Report (1886), p. 271. 1887.

[f] Lisfranc. Leçon sur l'Emploi du Muriate de Baryte contre les Tumeurs Blanches. Gaz. Méd. de Paris, 2 s., vol. 4, p. 215. 1836.

almost all recorded cases of locoed animals have occurred at a high altitude.

It must also be remembered that the addition of one salt to the solution of another may greatly increase the toxicity of the first one. Thus, the addition of a few milligrams of barium chlorid to a solution of a sulphocyanate renders the latter much more poisonous.[a] This may be due to the fact that the salts are more completely ionized.

PATHOLOGICAL LESIONS IN EXPERIMENTAL BARIUM POISONING.

The post-mortem examinations in cases of acute experimental barium poisoning, according to Schedel,[b] show punctiform or large hemorrhagic effusion in the fundus ventriculi[c] and in the large and small intestines, contraction of the bladder, and hemorrhage into the walls of the bladder and uterus. The heart is usually found relaxed or the left ventricle contracted in systole, while the right is relaxed. Only once were ecchymoses under the endocardium seen. The liver and kidneys showed nothing special. The urine was free from albumen and sugar. In a few cases the lungs showed some infiltration with blood. In chronic cases, according to our own investigations in rabbits, there are no characteristic macroscopic lesions, a result which agrees with Mittelstaedt's report.[d] Nothnagel and Rossbach[e] claim that in chronic poisoning by barium the peripheral nerves are altered. The same negative results have also been reported in chronic poisoning in higher animals. Reynolds[f] noted a layer like a blood clot under the cerebellum in a horse fed with barium chlorid. Fuchs[g] has called attention to the fact that the flesh of cattle poisoned with barium chlorid was harmless, perhaps owing to a conversion into an insoluble salt, a fact which may be considered in the use of locoed animals for food.

---

[a] Pauli, W., and Fröhlich, A. Pharmakodynam. Studien. Sitz. Kaiserl. Acad. d. Wissens. z. Wien, vol. 115, III, pt. 6, p. 445. 1906.

[b] Schedel, H. Beitr. z. Kennt. d. Wirkung des Chlorbariums. 1903, p. 13.

[c] After subcutaneous injection of barium chlorid, Lewin, by means of the spectroscope, has found barium in the stomach walls. Lewin, L. Schicksal körperfremder chem. Stoffe im Menschen u. besonders ihre Ausscheidung. Deutsch. Med. Woch., vol. 32, p. 173. 1906.

[d] Mittelstaedt, F. Ueber chronische Bariumvergiftung. Dissert., Greifswald, 1895, p. 29.

[e] Nothnagel, H., and Rossbach, M. J. Handb. d. Arzneimittel, p. 81. 1904.

[f] Reynolds, M. H. A Study of Certain Cathartics. Minn. Agric. Exper. Sta., 15th Ann. Rept. 1907.

[g] Fuchs, C. J. Vergiftungsfälle durch salzsäuren Baryt beim Rindvieh. Thierärztl. Mittheil., vol. 5, p. 159. 1870. Fuchs suggests that further investigations on this point are desirable. The literature of this class of experiments is very scanty. See Fröhner and Knudsen, Einige Versuche über d. Geniessbarkeit d. Fleisches vergift. Thiere. Monats. f. Prakt. Thierheilk., vol. 1, p. 529. 1890.

TOXICITY OF VARIOUS AQUEOUS EXTRACTS OF LOCO PLANTS.

On October 21, 1907, a rabbit weighing 1,531 grams was fed with an extract of 95 grams of dried *Aragallus lamberti* (Hugo, Colo., 1907), with an ash content of 12.44 per cent, with a barium content estimated as 2.6 milligrams of $BaSO_4$ in 1 gram of ash. On the following day it weighed 1,517 grams, and the same dose was again administered. On October 23 the weight was 1,488 grams, and the dose was repeated. On the next day the weight was the same and the dose was repeated. On October 26 the weight was 1,446 grams, and again the same extract was given. On October 30 the animal weighed 1,502.5 grams; on October 31, 1,531 grams. The animal received a total extract of 475 grams of the dried plant without serious injury. This result was apparently contradictory to the earlier work.

On October 21, 1907, a rabbit weighing 1,743 grams was fed with an extract of 47.5 grams of the same dried plant. On the next day its weight was 1,729 grams, and the same amount of the extract was fed. On October 23 the weight remained the same, and the dose was repeated. On October 24 the weight was 1,658 grams, and the same amount of extract was fed. On October 26 the animal weighed 1,630 grams, when it was again fed with the same amount of extract. On October 28 the animal weighed 1,573.5 grams, but two days later the weight had risen to 1,644 grams. An extract of 237.5 grams had been administered. Here again the results appeared contradictory.

On October 21, 1907, a rabbit weighing 1,517 grams was fed with an extract of 77.5 grams. On the next day it weighed 1,545 grams, and the dose was repeated. On October 23 the animal weighed 1,531 grams, and the same amount of extract was given. On the following day it weighed 1,488 grams, and the dose was repeated. On October 26 it weighed 1,474 grams, and again the dose was repeated. On October 30 the weight had risen to 1,545 grams, and on October 31 it was 1,559 grams. This animal received in all an extract of 387.5 grams of the dried plant. An aqueous extract of 200 grams of the same in one dose also failed to produce the acute symptoms.

These feeding experiments show little of the characteristic action seen in the earlier experiments made with aqueous extracts either of the dry plant or of the fresh plant preserved with chloroform. In other words, the aqueous extract of the dried plant was only slightly poisonous, yet the plant from which the extract was made contained barium.

Of this same dried loco 200 grams were then extracted with water and digested with pepsin and finally with pancreatin in the thermostat (37.5° C.). The extract was concentrated and fed to a rabbit weighing 1,616 grams. After five hours and ten minutes the animal appeared weak in the fore legs and unable to support himself, and he died during the night. The intestines the following morning were found full of gas, the stomach red, the lungs seemed normal, and the heart was relaxed.

A rabbit weighing 1,545 grams was fed on November 15, 1907, with a preparation made in a similar manner, save that the plant was not extracted with water before digestion. On the next day it weighed 1,517 grams and on November 19, 1,361 grams. The following day the weight was 1,318 grams; on November 21, 1,233 grams, and on the next day 1,162 grams. The animal died during the night, and the autopsy was made the following morning.

The animal was greatly emaciated and the subcutaneous fat had almost all disappeared. The mesenteric vessels were dilated, but the intestines were not dilated. The peritoneal cavity was normal. The kidneys were perhaps a little injected, and measured 3 cm. in length. The lungs were normal. The left ventricle was contracted and the rest of the heart relaxed. The liver was normal and the spleen apparently normal. The stomach walls were dark, owing to decomposition. No ulcers were seen. The suprarenals were perhaps a little enlarged. The examination of the brain was negative, and no clots were found.

A similar digestion from 200 grams of the same dried plant was then ashed and the ash treated with acetic acid and freed from acid by evaporation on the bath. The ash which was insoluble in water was ground up into a fine paste and the whole was fed to a rabbit weighing 992 grams. This animal died in forty minutes, showing the characteristic symptoms seen in acute cases already described. In the autopsy the lungs and other organs seemed perfectly normal macroscopically. The stomach walls, however, were reddened and ecchymotic, and the mesenteric vessels were dilated.

On January 8, 1908, a similar digestion of the same batch was treated with a few drops of sulphuric acid to remove the barium, and the filtrate was then treated with lead carbonate to remove the sulphuric acid. After careful filtering, H_2S was passed into the solution and after concentration was fed in one dose on January 9, 1908, to a rabbit. The following morning the rabbit had gained in weight. On January 14 this animal weighed 30 grams more than its initial weight.

The residue of this plant after such a digestion, examined by the Hillebrand method, showed no weighable amount of barium, so that it can be seen that barium in relatively large amount was found in the plant itself, but not after the digestion. It must therefore have been the aqueous digestion which produced the characteristic symptoms. The examination of this fluid for barium might, however, be misleading, as the large amount of proteids would unquestionably interfere with the determination of this amount of barium, unprotected by other salts and silica, so that this side of the investigation was not pursued. Control feedings with an emulsion of one-half gram each of pepsin and pancreatin proved inactive.

Of the same *Aragallus lamberti* 200 grams were similarly digested and the barium was removed with a few drops of H_2SO_4, the sulphuric acid by $PbCO_3$ and a little lead acetate, and the lead by H_2S. Such an extract it was shown in the previous experiment would not kill. However, to this extract was added 100 milligrams of crystallized barium acetate in a solution and a precipitate formed. Nevertheless, the liquid and the precipitate were fed on February 1, 1908, to a rabbit weighing 1,304 grams. On February 3 the animal weighed 1,233 grams; on February 4, 1,176 grams; February 5, 1,120 grams; February 6, 1,006 grams; February 7, 1,219 grams; February 8, 1,219 grams; February 10, 1,304 grams.

As a control for this animal, to make sure that the loss in weight was not due to the acetic acid set free by the treatment with H_2S, a similar aqueous extract of the same lot of *Aragallus lamberti* was precipitated with very much more lead acetate than in the preceding cases and also with lead subacetate and then H_2S. After evaporating to dryness this was fed on February 8, 1908, to a rabbit weighing 1,035 grams. On February 11 it weighed 1,021 grams; on February 13, 1,091 grams, and on February 15, 1,120 grams, showing a gain in weight.

Of the dried *Astragalus missouriensis* (Hugo, Colo., June, 1907) 400 grams with an ash content of 21.8 per cent and which was known to contain barium (3 mg. $BaSO_4$ in each 2 grams of the ash) were extracted with water and fed in four doses corresponding to 100 grams each in a period of four days. On November 18, 1907, the first day of feeding, this rabbit weighed 1,856.7 grams. Fifteen days later it weighed 1,984.3 grams.

One hundred grams of this dried plant after extraction with water were found to leave about 51.1 grams [a] of the plant undissolved. This when ashed yielded 8.2 grams of ash. Two grams of this ash yielded 5 milligrams of $BaSO_4$. In other words, the aqueous extract of the plant was inactive and the barium was found practically unextracted in the residue of the plant.

Evidently the barium in these dried plants had been converted into an insoluble form by drying or by some peculiarity of its metabolism, and was not extracted by water, but could be extracted by digesting the plants with the combined digestive ferments, pepsin and pancreatin.

---

[a] Some was lost, being attached to the cloth used in squeezing the extract.

Of the same dried *Astragalus missouriensis* 200 grams were extracted with water and the extract treated with lead carbonate to remove any possible free sulphates and after filtering this was treated with H$_2$S to remove the lead. As the preceding experiment showed that the aqueous extract of this dried plant was harmless without barium, the writer decided to add barium artificially, and 100 milligrams of barium phosphate,[a] crystallized, was added to the liquid and the whole fed to a rabbit weighing 2,423.9 grams. The following morning the rabbit was found dead. The autopsy was made by Dr. H. J. Washburn, of the Bureau of Animal Industry. He found that the suprarenals were enlarged and congested, and there were small areas of hepatization at the apex of each lung. There were also acute corrosion areas on the greater curvature of the stomach and over the upper portion of the duodenum.

Of the *Astragalus missouriensis* used in the preceding experiments, 200 grams were extracted thoroughly with water, and the extract corresponding to 100 grams, together with 80 milligrams of barium phosphate pure, was fed on March 12, 1908, to a rabbit weighing 1,261.5 grams. During this day the animal walked at times with an uncertain gait and the following morning it weighed 1,233 grams. It was then fed the rest of the solution, that is, the extract of the remaining 100 grams of the plant, but without any barium. The animal soon developed convulsions and died in a little over twenty-four hours after the original feeding. The autopsy, which was made by Dr. J. R. Mohler, of the Bureau of Animal Industry, showed that the mucous membrane of the stomach was markedly hemorrhagic and in areas gelatinous infiltration was very marked. In one portion of this hemorrhagic area there was distinct erosion. The large intestines were full of gas, the lungs were normal, the heart was relaxed, and the lungs collapsed. The blood vessels of the kidneys were markedly engorged.

Of the dried *Astragalus nitidus* (Woodland Park, Colo., October, 1907) which was reported by the Bureau of Chemistry as containing no barium, 200 grams were extracted with water and fed in 100-gram doses for two successive days. The animal increased steadily in weight and fifteen days after the first feeding had gained 99.2 grams. This amount of the plant was also extracted with water and the residue was then digested with pepsin and pancreatin in the thermostat, as in the previous case, and fed in two doses corresponding to 100 grams each. This animal increased in weight, gaining 60 grams in six days and 165 grams in addition after a further fifteen days.

---

[a] This barium phosphate was determined by the Bureau of Chemistry to be BaHPO$_4$ and to contain traces of iron, sodium, and potassium, but it was free from arsenic.

An *Astragalus mollissimus* (Kit Carson County, Colo., December, 1906), which was also reported by the Bureau of Chemistry as containing no barium, was extracted with water, and a dose corresponding to an extract of 200 grams of the dried plant was fed in one dose without any serious result. The same amount of the dried plant was also similarly digested with pepsin and pancreatin and fed in two doses, but without the production of any symptoms, the rabbit gaining 60 grams in four days.

Of the *Aragallus lamberti* (Hugo, Colo., June, 1907), with an ash content of 12.44 per cent, 250 grams were ashed and the ash treated with acetic acid and, after evaporating off the acetic acid, was extracted with water and the ash digested with pepsin and pancreatin. The aqueous extract and the digestion products of the ash were then fed after concentration, but without any serious effects to the animal, indicating that in this plant the barium is in a form insoluble in water and in the ashing is further changed so that it can not now be made soluble by digestion—an opposite result to the experiment in which the barium was first rendered soluble by digestion and the digestion products ashed, suggesting a possibility that plants might be found in which the barium is not extracted by digestion, at present a hypothesis.

Of dried *Astragalus decumbens* (Ephraim, Utah, 1907), which was reported by the Bureau of Chemistry to contain no barium, 200 grams also failed to produce symptoms in rabbits by our test.

A solution containing 50 milligrams of barium acetate (crystallized) was mixed with an aqueous extract of 200 grams of the dried *Aragallus lamberti* which had proved inactive pharmacologically, but a precipitate formed ($BaSO_4$?) and the extract still remained inactive, suggesting that the question of toxicity depended not only upon the presence of barium, but also whether other agents, such as sulphates, etc., might not be present in sufficient amount to render the barium insoluble; that is, pharmacologically inactive.

This *Aragallus lamberti* yielded an ash content of 37.3 per cent, and the SO_3 group was estimated at 0.27 per cent of the ash, while a corresponding lot which was obtained two years later from the same area yielded an ash content of 12.44 per cent and a SO_3 content of 0.24 per cent of the ash.

It may be urged that the full lethal dose of the barium was not always found in the plant, yet it must be remembered that the toxic action was the resultant of the action of the total constituents and that if the barium was removed the extract was practically harmless.

In looking back over the work the most suitable preparation for producing the characteristic symptoms in rabbits seems to be the freshly ground-up plant mixed with water and preserved in chloroform, for while the dried plant might contain barium, yet the aqueous extract was often inactive, suggesting, perhaps, the presence of something in the fresh plant which aided the solution of the barium, thus accounting for the variations in toxicity of aqueous extracts made from plants dried under varying conditions. The nature of the compound in which barium exists in the plant is as yet unknown and has not been investigated. *It is important to remember that not only must barium be found in the plant to prove poisonous, but it must be in such a form that it can be extracted in the gastro-intestinal canal.*

The amount of barium found in various species of loco plants will no doubt vary, and perhaps the pharmacological test on rabbits as the writer has used it may have to be modified for such plants, so that at present the wisest plan to test these plants is to determine their barium content and also make the physiological test, as has been proposed, and if the barium content runs low, say below 0.11 per cent of the ash, in plants yielding from 12 to 18 per cent of ash, then to increase the number of feedings on the rabbit. No doubt on ranges where a large number of loco plants are eaten, with little other food, plants with a very low barium content may be poisonous, but if large amounts of other food are fed the writer would expect few, if any, serious results.

As the writer's work has been confined to the laboratory side of the loco-weed investigations no feeding experiments with barium salts have been made by him on large animals. Such experiments should, of course, be made under range conditions; that is, where the water and food supply is deficient.

THEORETICAL ANTIDOTE FOR LOCO-WEED POISONING.

The fact that treatment of the loco-weed extract with a few drops of sulphuric acid, which will remove the barium, renders these extracts harmless, and even apparently nutritious, would suggest the theoretical antidotal treatment to be with sulphates, in the form, perhaps, of epsom salts, but perhaps alkaline bicarbonates may be present in the stomach, either due to lessened acidity of the stomach or from drinking alkaline waters, in which case the precipitation of the barium by sulphates would presumably be interfered with, and thus the treatment be rendered ineffectual.[a] It is interesting to note that most of the remedies proposed for the successful treatment of locoed animals contain sulphates.[b]

In Storer's experiments on feeding rats with barium carbonate it was found that the barium carbonate would kill them, but if calcium carbonate was mixed with the barium the rats survived, sug-

---

[a] Mendel, L. B., and Sicher, D. F., l. c., p. 148.

[b] Mayo, N. S. Some Observations upon Loco. Kans. State Agric. Coll. Bul. 35, p. 119. 1893.

gesting an antidotal action. This apparent antagonism deserves further study and may lead to practical results.[a] A somewhat similar antagonism for at least a part of the action of barium has been claimed to exist between barium and potassium.[b] However, extracts of ashed plants, treated with acetic acid, which contained calcium and potassium, caused death in the experiments of the writer, but no work has yet been done by him as to the antidotal action of calcium carbonate on barium. Then, too, as Lüdeking[c] pointed out, large quantities of calcium chlorid may interfere with the precipitation of barium as a sulphate. It is well known that the presence of various salts influences the solubility of barium sulphate in water,[d] and the fact that barium has been found in solution in the urine in the presence of sulphates shows that the precipitation of barium as a sulphate in the body is not so simple as in test-tube experiments.[e] Again, in very dilute solutions, such as must necessarily occur at any one time in the stomach, the precipitate with sulphates only slowly forms and the barium may be absorbed before the insoluble compound can be formed.[f] Evidently an important point to be considered in the antidotal treatment of locoed animals with sulphates is the possibility of inducing a gastritis, with its attendant loss of weight. It therefore seems apparent that the proper treatment at present is preventive—that is, removal from the plants.

Lewin[g] has suggested the possibility of acquiring some immunity to barium, but our experiments point against the production of any practical immunity.

ACTION OF BARIUM ON DOMESTIC AND FARM ANIMALS.

Barium in the form of barium chlorid has been recently introduced into veterinary therapeutics by Dieckerhoff[h] in the treatment of

---

[a] Storer, F. H. Experiments on Feeding Mice with Painter's Putty and with Other Mixtures of Pigments and Oils. Bul. of Bussey Institute, vol. 2, p. 274. 1884.

[b] Brunton, T. L., and Cash, J. T. Contribution to Our Knowledge of the Connection between Chemical Constitution, Physiological Action, and Antagonism. Philos. Trans. Royal Soc. London, I, vol. 175, p. 229. 1884.

[c] Lüdeking, C. Analyse d. Barytgruppe. Zelts. f. Anal. Chem., vol. 29, p. 556. 1890.

[d] Fraps, G. S. Solubility of Barium Sulphate in Ferric Chloride, Aluminum Chloride, and Magnesium Chloride. Amer. Chem. Journ., vol. 27, p. 288. 1902.

[e] Santi has paid special attention to the solubility of barium in the body.

[f] Fresenius, C. G. Man. of Qualitat. Chem. Anal. Tr. by H. L. Wells, 1904, p. 148.

[g] Lewin, L. Nebenwirkungen d. Arzneimittel, 2 ed., p. 439. 1893.

[h] Dieckerhoff. Ueber d. Wirkung d. Chlorbaryum bei Pferden, Rindern und Schafen. Berliner Thierärztl. Woch., p. 265; see also pp. 313 and 337, 1895; Abstract in Vet. Mag., vol. 2, p. 360. 1895.

constipation, but Winslow [a] says that " the doses required to produce catharsis in the horse are almost toxic," and he advises against the intravenous use of this remedy.

Fröhner [b] has carefully summarized the literature on the use of barium chlorid in veterinary work, and reports that its use in the Zürich clinic has recently been so unsatisfactory that it is now seldom employed and that in the last ten years the preponderance of reports in the literature are unfavorable to the use of this agent in colic.

After the administration per os, much of the barium must be carried off in the diarrheal stools. A number of deaths in horses have been attributed to the use of this agent. No doubt the presence of sulphates, etc., derived from the food would render the barium insoluble in the gastro-intestinal tract, and this would explain the lack of poisonous action in certain of the cases in which large doses of barium proved harmless.

Husard and Biron administered daily doses of 8 grams of barium chlorid to one horse, and the same amount of barium carbonate to a second horse, for several days. A fortnight later the first horse unexpectedly died, and the second a few days later. The post-mortem examination was negative.[c] A third horse fed with barium carbonate also died suddenly. Recently barium occurring in brine has given rise to acute poisoning in stock.[d]

In a case reported by Stietenroth [e] the horse died after the injection of 0.5 gram of barium chlorid into the jugular vein. A number of sudden deaths in horses after the intravenous injection of 0.7 gram and over of barium chlorid have been collected by Fröhner.[f] The lethal dose by mouth for acute poisoning with barium chlorid in horses lies between 8 to 12 grams, while cattle require much larger doses (40 grams)[g] to induce death.

Dieckerhoff advises against the use of barium chlorid in the treatment of constipation in sheep.

---

[a] Winslow, K. Vet. Materia Medica and Therapeutics, p. 152. 1901.

[b] Fröhner, E. Lehrb. d. Arzneimittellehre, p. 399. 1906. Fröhner gives a detailed account of these cases.

Original note in Ehrhardt, J. Erfahrungen ü. ältere u. neue Arzneimittel. Schweizer Archiv. f. Thierheilk., vol. 41, p. 44. 1899.

[c] Pelletier. Observations on Strontian. Journ. Nat. Philos., vol. 1, p. 529. 1797; original in Annales de Chimie, vol. 21, p. 127. 1797.

[d] Howard, C. D. Occurrence of Barium in the Ohio Valley Brines and Its Relation to Stock Poisoning. W. Va. Univ. Agric. Exper. Sta. Bul. 103. 1906.

[e] Stietenroth. Ueber Chlorbarium bei der Kolik der Pferde. Berliner Thierärztl. Woch., p. 16. 1899.

[f] Fröhner, E. Lehrb. d. Toxikol., 2 ed., p. 116. 1901.

[g] Fröhner, E., l. c., p. 116.

See similar reports in Veterinarian, vol. 68, p. 572, 1895, and vol. 69, p. 228, 1896; Zeits. f. Veterinärk., vol. 8, pp. 99 and 211, 1896; Nagler, F., Berliner Thierärztl. Woch., p. 65. 1896.

After a dose of 6 grams of barium chlorid a 2-year-old healthy ram appeared perfectly well, but the following day he was depressed, refused to eat, staggered, and became so weak that he was unable to stand. The muscles of the extremities were paralyzed and the animal died. " The post-mortem examination revealed œdema of the lungs, slight cloudiness of the heart muscles, numerous small hemorrhagic spots on the mucous membrane of the small intestine, and stagnation of the blood in the vessels of the small and large intestines. Similar symptoms and lesions were found in a lamb 4 months old which was given per os 6.0 grams of barium chlorid dissolved in 200 grams of distilled water." [a]

Poisonings with barium carbonate have also been reported in pigs.[b] Domestic animals pastured in the neighborhood of barite deposits soon succumb,[c] and accidental cases of poisoning are reported in cows. Poisoning in dogs has also been reported after the subcutaneous use of this agent.[d] Linossier says that if the barium salts are used for any time the salts are deposited in various organs, largely in the kidneys, brain, and medulla, but especially in the bones.[e]

APPLICATION OF THE RESULTS OF THESE INVESTIGATIONS TO THE RANGE.

It has been calculated that a medium estimate of food for cattle on green fodder is about 60 pounds (30 kilos) a day.[f] Calculating this entirely in terms of *Aragallus lamberti* and allowing 10 per cent of moisture for these plants (Sayre) would make 27 kilos of dry loco

---

[a] Dieckerhoff, W. Vet. Mag., vol. 2, p. 362. 1895.

[b] Kabitz, H. Ueber d. Wirkung einiger Baryumsalze beim Schwein. Deutsch. Thierärztl. Woch., vol. 13, p. 317. 1905.

[c] Parkes. Chem. Essays, vol. 2, p. 213. Quoted by Christison, R., in Treatise on Poisons, Edinburgh, 4 ed., p. 581, 1845.—Fuchs, C. J. Vergiftungsfälle durch salzsäuren Baryt beim Rindvieh. Thierärztl. Mittheil., vol. 5, pp. 133, 154. 1870.

[d] Falk. Zur Vergift. von Hunden mit Chlorbarium. Berliner Thierärztl. Woch., p. 40. 1897.—Schirmer, Chlorbariumvergift. beim Hunde. Berliner Thierärztl. Woch., vol. 23, p. 268. 1897.

[e] Linossier, G. De la Localisation du Baryum dans l'Organisme à la Suite de l'Intoxication Chronique par un Sel de Baryum. Comp. Rend. Hebd. Soc. de Biol., 8 s., vol. 4, p. 123. 1887.

NOTE.—Other cases of poisoning in animals may be found in Marder, Beitrag z. Giftwirkung des Baryum chloratum. Berliner Thierärztl. Woch., vol. 37, p. 436. 1897; Absichtliche Vergift. mit Chlorbarium. Zeits. f. Veterinärk., vol. 9, p. 72. 1897.

[f] Lane, C. B. Soiling Crop Experiments. N. J. Agric. Exper. Sta. Bul. 158, p. 18. 1902.—Woll, F. W. One Hundred American Rations for Dairy Cows. Univ. Wis. Agric. Exper. Sta. Bul. 38, p. 12. 1894.—N. J. State Agric. Exper. Sta., 20th Ann. Rept. (1899), p. 193. 1900.

eaten by each animal per diem. In the analysis of the writer of one *Aragallus lamberti* from Hugo, Colo., it was found to yield 12.44 per cent of ash, and the barium content corresponded to 2.6 milligrams $BaSO_4$ in each gram of the ash. This would correspond to 10.24 grams of barium acetate $(Ba(C_2H_3O_2)_2 + H_2O)$ or 9.15 grams of barium chlorid $(BaCl_2 + 2H_2O)$ per diem. This amount daily administered would, theoretically, readily produce chronic poisoning owing to the accumulation in the system, as was shown in the case of rabbits.

There is, however, some question as to whether this full theoretical amount of loco plants is eaten on the range, and the estimate has been made that one-sixth of this amount only would be actually taken. It must be remembered, as Stalker pointed out, that locoed animals develop an especial taste for these plants and after a time reject other food, so that while the number of loco plants at first taken may be small, yet later, perhaps, it is greater. A part of this barium, however, may not be taken up by the system, but may pass out undissolved. No actual experiments have yet been made with cattle by feeding small doses of the pure salt.

No doubt more of the pure barium salts will be required to produce symptoms of poisoning in animals than would be necessary in the case of the form of barium found in the plant, as in the loco weed the barium is probably better protected from precipitation than are the barium salts when dissolved in water alone.

CONCLUSIONS.[a]

(1) Conditions analogous to those met with in locoed animals occur in other portions of the world, especially Australia.

(2) The main symptoms described in stock on the range can be reproduced on rabbits by feeding extracts of certain loco plants. Those especially referred to here under the term "loco plants" are *Astragalus mollissimus* and *Aragallus lamberti*.

(3) The production of chronic symptoms in rabbits is a crucial test of the pharmacological activity of these plants.

(4) The inorganic constituents, especially barium, are responsible for this action, at least in the plants collected at Hugo, Colo. Perhaps in other portions of the country other poisonous principles may be found.

---

[a] Résumé of the results of the loco-weed investigations carried on by the Bureau of Plant Industry was issued as Bulletin 121, part 3, Bureau of Plant Industry, on January 28, 1908, in the form of papers by C. Dwight Marsh and Albert C. Crawford, respectively, under the titles "Results of Loco-Weed Investigations in the Field" and "Laboratory Work on Loco-Weed Investigations."

(5) A close analogy exists between the clinical symptoms and pathological findings in barium poisoning and those resulting from feeding extracts of certain loco plants. Small doses of barium salts may be administered to rabbits without apparent effect, but suddenly acute symptoms set in analogous to what is reported on the range.

(6) The administration of sulphates, especially epsom salts, to form insoluble barium sulphate would be the chemical antidote which would logically be inferred from the laboratory work, but of necessity this would have to be frequently administered and its value after histological changes in the organs have occurred remains to be settled. But even the treatment of acute cases of barium poisoning in man is not always successful, even when sulphates combined with symptomatic treatment are employed. The conditions under which the sulphates fail to precipitate barium must be considered. At present it seems best to rely on preventive measures rather than on antidotal treatment.

(7) Loco plants grown on certain soils are inactive pharmacologically and contain no barium. In drying certain loco plants the barium apparently is rendered insoluble so that is is not extracted by water, but can usually be extracted by digestion with the digestive ferments.

(8) The barium to be harmful must be in such a form as to be dissolved out by digestion.

(9) In deciding whether plants are poisonous it is desirable not merely to test the aqueous or alcoholic extract, but also the extracts obtained by digesting these plants with the ferments which occur in the gastro-intestinal tract.

(10) It is important that the ash of plants, especially those grown on uncultivated soil, as on our unirrigated plains, be examined for various metals, using methods similar to those by which rocks are now analyzed in the laboratory of the United States Geological Survey.

(11) It is desirable to study various obscure chronic conditions, such as lathyrism, with a view to determine the inorganic constituents of lathyrus and other families of plants.

129

INDEX.

O

CPSIA information can be obtained
at www.ICGtesting.com
Printed in the USA
BVHW071627280119
538839BV00028B/2175/P